3

NURSE

Other books by William H. Hull

ALL HELL BROKE LOOSE

THE DIRTY THIRTIES

NURSE

Hearts and Hands

Nurses Tell Their Most
Memorable Events

by

William H. Hull, M.A.

This book
is dedicated
to all the nurses
whose actions say they agree
with this statement by Thomas Carlyle:

"It is the heart always that sees,
before the head can see."*

*"Chartism", 1893

CONTENTS

NURSE

NURSE

INTRODUCTION

As I sit here on Thanksgiving day while Carol stuffs the bird, my thoughts go to the hundreds of nurses with whom I've had contact in my life.

The first contact was in St. Joseph's Catholic hospital in Boonville, Missouri where this ten year old boy had undergone an appendectomy and was sick from ether. These nurses were Benedictine sisters who dressed in long, flowing white outfits except for a few that were entirely in black, like the mourning ladies at my brother's funeral just two years previously. They were scary, these tall penguins of such formidable appearance.

Ah, but they were all angels of mercy. And I soon learned to love them for the love they extended to me.

Nurses have come a long way since then, baby. Oh, boy, have they come a long way. In some hospitals one can't find the prototyped nurse in white dress and white cap. In the large hospital where I work as a volunteer, each department has developed its own color scheme for dress. There are pale blues, there are dark blues, some greens, some scrubs, one group wears flowered outfits. Each wants to have its own identity. Does it make one more proud to be part of the group? Or is it that one wants to avoid being categorized with another less prestigious group?

No, I think it is due to specialization. A pediatric nurse, a surgical nurse, an oncology nurse has each received special training and each is proud to be so identified. An emergency room nurse is trained to meet special situations and probably wants the world to know that she works in ER. A cardiac special care nurse has exactly the same situation. After receiving that special training and after working in that special area she has something that just any old nurse doesn't have—and she's proud to be so identified.

So, maybe, after all, it's a matter of ego.

I'm convinced that the disappeared nurse's cap was lost to ego.

Some nurses feel that the cap was a symbol of servitude, an indication of a minor league rating that has outlived its usefulness. When they were capped and pinned years ago it was a meaningful moment but in the real world it meant taking orders and doing little on their own initiative.

In the meantime nurses have been permitted greater latitude for judgement. Many have taken advanced degrees—as I mentioned —to specialize in treatment in a special area. Many have become Physician's Assistants, a whole new category that recognizes special ability and experience. We talk to them many times, not realizing that they are PAs. They will consult with us regarding medication changes and dosages and perform many routine assignments which a nurse of 20 years ago would have been kicked out the door for doing.

I respect today's nurses. As a class I have a great love for them. They have been by my side several times when I needed someone badly. When admitted to ER with a split skull, there was a great nurse to soothe my wounded spirit and to help the MD who sewed up my wounds. When recovering from one of several following surgeries there was a whole battery of nurses dedicated to make me well. When I lay in my bed for a month wearing a halo ring, there was a special nurse who, even though not assigned to me, would slip into my room to console and/or visit with me. I can't forget that little Filipino lady who took me as a personal friend and guaranteed that I got all the attention I could stand. I can't forget the nurses who saw me through a heart attack during that same period— lovely, caring people who were giving their whole lives to people like me.

When I was as well as I was ever going to be and started volunteering in another big hospital, one of the first nurses I met was Kit, a senior ER nurse. It was Kit who taught me how to wash my hands, turning off the water with a towel rather than redirtying my hands from any contaminant I might have placed on the handles when turning them on. It was Kit who encouraged my desire to be warm and friendly to incoming patients. It was Kit whom I took as a role model.

Every week I see some amazing performances by nurses—and no one will ever criticize them to me without receiving a full lecture.

NURSE

They are some of the world's most gracious people, working long variable hours, underpaid, maybe thanked too infrequently, but still dedicated to helping you and me. Thanks, Virginia. Thanks, Kit. Thanks, Peg. Thanks, Dorothea. Thanks from all of us who are alive and better because of you.

William H. Hull, MA

SHE SPEAKS FOR ME

The nurse's role in the physician's office has changed gradually and dramatically, a change for which we should be thankful. No longer is she/he just a minor assistant permitted to bandage a small wound or administer a pill—she is now more frequently a top assistant, perhaps even a junior physician for lack of a better term.

She frequently writes prescriptions, which the doctor has ordered, and probably takes to him for signature. She has many increasingly important responsibilities.

Why not? When a highly qualified, trained assistant in almost any other field is used intelligently it is to relieve the prime person of routine responsibilities. Hence a physician can make very good utilization of his nurse assistant.

This sometimes gets carried to the sublime ridiculous. In some offices the nurse acts as a buffer; she becomes the locked door beyond which the patient cannot go with ease. At the greatest extreme she becomes the aggressive questioner who requests more confidentiality than the patient wants to impart. Thus a testy confrontation between nurse and patient could occur.

This part of the nurse's role seems to work best when she/he serves as a consultant and message carrier. She reviews the situation with the patient, by telephone in many cases, and relays the information to the physician. Then she returns to the patient with a report and plan of treatment. This can relieve the physician of considerable work, yet it also can insulate him from the patient. It can make the patient believe the physician has no interest in him.

If that is the procedure in an office it probably works best when the physician either returns the patient call personally or when the nurse uses such expressions as "Doctor Jones asked me to tell you . . ."

Of course the very bad situation occurs when the patient never hears from anyone after having made the initial call.

4

How does the patient feel when a nurse makes the treatment decision—in lieu of the physician doing so? He/she is probably not too pleased. After all, he thinks, it is the physician to whom he's paid fees, the physician who has a financial/patient obligation to respond. If handled carefully, this situation can only enhance the nurse's position because the patient sees that the doctor has faith in her. Maybe the physician should even inform his patients that "she speaks for me." That, of course, can become a legally awkward situation.

No patient wants to be treated flippantly and the nurse is not apt to do so. When I witness a nurse substituting for an unavailable physician, I glory in it and accept the recommendation. Obviously the physician permits her to take that authority in his office. Hence the nurse has again helped upgrade her profession in the public eye.

FROM HER CAME NURSING

"On February 7, 1837, God spoke to me and called me to His service." Thus spoke Florence Nightingale, the founder of nursing, who then spent most of her life trying to identify what God wanted from her.[1]

Florence had been born May 12, 1820, of wealthy British parents, Fanny and William Nightingale, while they were touring Europe. In fact, it was in Florence, Italy, where our Florence was born and got her name.

Florence was "a charming and gifted young daughter, destined for a brilliant social success. She was graceful, witty, vividly good looking. Her hair was of an unusual beauty, bright chestnut in color, thick, glossy and wavy. In middle age her hair became dark but at nineteen it was golden-red."[2]

But throughout her life she had problems, always wondering why and how she was not like other children, being "afraid to meet strangers, particularly children" and thinking she might be some sort of monster.[3]

Always interested in mathematics, as a young girl she studied it very seriously. In a different era she probably would have become a noted mathematician, perhaps a physicist.

By the time she was in her mid twenties she began to realize that her future lay with disadvantaged people, particularly those in hospitals. She found an increasing interest in helping the sick, working with the ill within her own family.

It must be remembered that these were Victorian years when wealthy ladies such as her mother, busied themselves almost solely with social entertaining. Of course no lady would even consider working in a hospital. In fact there is little indication that the gentry ever were treated in hospitals, their care probably being given at home.

Neither Florence "nor anyone she had ever met had been taught how to nurse. It was universally assumed that the only qualification needed for taking care of the sick, was to be a woman."[4]

Eventually, Florence wanted to go to the Salisbury Infirmary for a three-month basic training in health. When she proposed her plan to her family "a storm burst. Mama was terrified. Parthe (her sister) got hysterics. Florence persisted and her mother's terror passed into furious anger. In floods of tears Fanny (mother) wept that Florence wanted to disgrace herself."[5]

The mother's opposition to this move can be understood when existing conditions are remembered. "Hospitals were places of wretchedness, degradation, and squalor. 'Hospital smell,' the result of dirt and lack of sanitation, was acceptable as unavoidable. Wards were usually large, bare and gloomy. Beds were crammed in, fifty or sixty, less thatn two feet apart. Even decency was impossible. Fifteen years later, *when improvements had been made*, (Editor's italics.) Florence wrote in 'Notes on Hospitals:' 'The floors were made of ordinary wood which, owing to lack of cleaning and lack of sanitary conveniences for the patients' use, had become saturated with organic matter, which, when washed, gave off the smell of something quite different from soap and water. Walls and ceilings were of common plaster, also saturated with impurity. Heating was supplied by a single fire at the end of each ward and in winter windows were kept closed for warmth, sometimes for months at a time. In some hospitals half the windows were boarded up in winter. After a time the smell became sickening, walls streamed with moisture and a 'minute vegetation appeared.' The remedy for this was frequent lime washing and scraping, but the workmen engaged on the task frequently became seriously ill.' "[6]

So Florence Nightingale really deserves the accolade of being the Mother of Nursing.

She wanted to do so much for other people that she even put together a booklet named "Notes on Nursing" to help people giving home care to their families. In the preface, she said:

"The following notes are by no means intended as a rule of thought by which nurses can teach themselves to nurse, still less as a manual to teach nurses to nurse . . . I do not pretend to teach her how, I ask her to teach herself, and for this purpose I venture to give her some hints."[7]

". . . nursing as a handicraft, has not been treated of here for three reasons: 1. that these notes do not pretend to be a manual for nursing, any more than for cooking for the sick; 2. that the writer, who has herself seen more of what may be called surgical nursing, i.e., practical manual nursing, than, perhaps, anyone in Europe, honestly believes that it is impossible to learn it from any book, and that it can only be thoroughly learnt in the wards of a hospital; and she also honestly believes that the perfection of surgical nursing may be seen practised by the old-fashioned "Sister" of a London hospital, as it can be seen nowhere else in Europe. 3. While thousands die of foul air, etc., who have this surgical nursing to perfection, the converse is comparatively rare."

Nightingale's "little book of notes" truly is a discussion of many facets of home healthcare. In these 79 pages she discusses such mundane subjects as the sick person's diet, feeding the patient who can't take food, the importance of providing a quiet atmosphere, *ad infinitum*. It's impressing just to read a few lines about caring for bed and bedding:

"If you consider that an adult in health exhales by the lungs and skin in the twenty-four hours three pints at least of moisture, loaded with organic matter ready to enter into putrefaction; that in sickness the quantity is often greatly increased, the quality is always more noxious—just ask youself next where does all this moisture go to? Chiefly into the bedding, because it cannot go anywhere else. And it stays there; because, perhaps, a weekly change of sheets, scarcely any other airing is attempted. A nurse will be careful to fidgetiness about airing the clean sheets from clean damp, but airing the dirty sheets from noxious damp will never even occur to her. Besides this, the most dangerous effluvia we know of are from the excreta of the sick—these are placed, at least temporarily, where they must throw their effluvia into the under side of the bed, and the space under the bed is never aired. . . . Must not such a bed be always saturated, and be always the means of re-introducing into the system of the unfortunate patient who lives in it, that excrementitious matter to eliminate which from the body nature had expressly appointed the disease."[9]

1. "Lonely Crusader, The Life of Florence Nightingale," by Cecil Woodham-Smith, Bantam Books, New York, February 1963. First published as "Florence Nightingale," McGraw-Hill, New York, 1951. Page 19.

2. Ibid, p. 19.

3. Ibid, p. 4.

4. Ibid, p. 32.

5. Ibid, p. 32.

6. Ibid, p. 34.

7. "Notes on Nursing," by Florence Nightingale, Brandon Systems Press, Inc., 1970 printing, London, "For the Labouring Classes." Page: Preface.

8. Ibid, pp. 71, 72.

9. Ibid. p. 45.

Editor's postscript: Over a period of a year we made great effort to determine copyright of "Lonely Crusader" or "Florence Nightingale," and to obtain reprint permission. This included several overseas telephone calls, but no one would claim copyright. A year of fourteen different contacts failed. Each firm referred us to another. Among those contacted were, in this sequence: Penguin Books, New York; Bantam Books, New York; McGraw-Hill, New York; Hamish-Hamilton, London; Constable Publishing, London; HarperCollins, New York; Graw-Hill, New York (second reference); and Hamish-Hamilton, London (second reference).

EVERY SOLDIER'S OLD MAID AUNT

The Angel of the Battlefield was the nickname given Clara Barton, the founder of the American Red Cross, and probably the person who did more for nursing than any other non-nurse in modern history. It might be most correct to refer to her as an humanitarian and to remember that Civil War soldiers dubbed her "every soldier's old maid aunt."[1]

Before leaving for the front to join the army near Fredericksburg, Virginia, Clara Barton visited her family in Massachusetts. Then she headed for the army, where her medical stores were enthusiastically received. Later, back in Washington, she heard of a big battle between the two armies near Culpepper, Virginia, with Union casualties being about 2,000. So, she stepped into the breach and went to the fighting.

This should give us an idea of what Clara did, how she worked supplying hospitals with basic items. Doctors were out of bandages; there were needs so basic that everything she supplied was put to immediate and grateful use. Dr. James Dunn, a Pennsylvania surgeon, later wrote to his wife "I thought that night, if heaven ever sent out a homely angel, she must be one; her assistance was so timely."

"At the main street hospital and at countless private houses. . . she saw that the anguished men covered the bare floors, lying in their own blood and filth, some without arms and legs, others with jaws or hands blown away. Many of the wounded had lain on the field in the blistering sun until a flag of truce allowed them to be cleared off. Sunstroke, dehydration and shock increased their suffering. When thanking the women who had sent boxes of cooling cordials and soft linen shirts, she could write: 'You will believe they were welcome when I tell you that we put shirts on men who had been stripped on the field and lain with naked breast in the scorching sun two days.' "[2]

She served at many battlefields; tales are told of her at the Second Battle of Bull Run near Manassas, at Harper's Ferry, at South Mountain. Everywhere, she went to the men to aid and relieve their pain, to see that they had a drink of water, that they were as comfortable as possible when being transported. As she got closer and closer to combat, as she was immediately behind the cannons, where she wanted to be, she encountered scenes to burn themselves into her memory.

For example, "the fighting was barely over when she arrived at the battlefield (at South Mountain). Almost more dreadful than she could contemplate, the sight merited the only description she would write of a field of war. It was 'all blood and carnage,' she wrote with revulsion, 'our wagon wheels within six feet of unburied dead. A mingled mass of stiffened, blackened men, horses, muskets, bayonets, knapsacks, haversacks, blankets, coats, canteens, broken wheels and cannon balls which had done this deadly work—the very earth plowed with shot . . . It was a painful way to learn of a battle, a hard page to read.' She and Welles (her assistant) 'shocked and sick at heart,' climbed over the hills and ledges to find the last wounded man and see that he got medical attention, then trod through the field to answer screams and whimpers. The last she saw of 'that field of death' was the lingering haze of smoke and a 'hideous pile of mangled and dismembered bodies.' "[3] (Clara Barton to Ladies of the Soldiers' Friend Society of Hightstown, N.J., February 14, 1863, newspaper clipping in Clara Barton Scrapbook, in the Library of Congress).

She was at Antietam Creek where she "cut an eccentric figure, standing over a kettle of gruel, with the hem of her skirt pinned up about her waist, her hair astray, her face covered with gunpowder. But no surgeon would have thought to laugh at the sight. She had the habit of command and comfort, and the soldier aides turned naturally to her for instructions, which she always gave in a calm and infuriatingly unhurried manner. When, exhausted from the unrelieved misery, the medical men denounced the indifferent government that left them to cope in the dark without a single candle, she gently told them of the candles and lanterns she had brought. She would not flinch as she held a leg that had to be hacked off without chloroform, did not cry at the ghastly death of some former pupil. 'Now what do you think of Miss Barton?' Surgeon Dunn asked his wife, after describing to her some of these feats. 'In my feeble estimation, General McClellan, with all his laurels, sinks into insignifance beside the true heroine of the age, *the angel of the battlefield,*' "[4] quoting from "Dunn to wife, undated clipping, Clara Barton Papers, Manuscript Division, Library of Congress, Washington, D.C.")

So now, Clara Barton had her sobriquet—"The Angel of the Battlefield."

In 1855 she had been working as a clerk in the Patent Office in Washington, one of four female clerks, all about to be relieved because a superior thought men should have those jobs. The entire department was in such a confused stage that an attempt was being made to unravel it, and Clara helped pinpoint some of the people who were selling patent privileges illegally. Of course she was then unpopular and her "own reputation for lax sexual conduct during this period was probably based more on the boldness of her employment than any real promiscuity."[5]

The Patent Office work was demanding and exhausting. "An examiner complained that he had to get to the office at 5:00 A.M. to make any headway on his work load. Barton was copying over a thousand pages a month of 'dry lawyer writing' into a ledger too heavy for her to lift. "My arm is tired," she told her sister-in-law, Julia Barton, "and my poor thumb is all calloused holding my pen." But she was making money and accumulating some for a change.[6]

Her work in the Civil War really started in Washington when she was interviewed by a Colonel Rucker whom she told she wanted to go to the front. Of course he demurred with the speech of that's-no-place-for-a-lady. "But with a studied meekness she told him she only wanted to distribute some stores she had collected for the soldiers. She needed a pass and some wagons. Then she played her final card, telling him this was no basket of made-by-loving-hand delicacies she was describing, but three warehouses full of hospital stores and food—everything, in fact, that the soldiers needed. In an instant Barton's life changed. With a haste that seemed absurd in light of the months of tedious waiting, Rucker wrote out an order for six wagons, teamsters, and men to load them, and requests to the surgeon general, secretary of war, military governor of Washington, D.C., and other crucial officers to allow (her) to pass through the lines.

She was back "in Washington in 1863 where the Union army had settled into sluggish inactivity. She wore her shabby dress with pride, feeling it was one more link between her and her tattered foot soldiers. Her financial condition was so bad that she depended on the army and personal friends for basic food and army rations. Her tattered clothes caught the attention of friends in Worcester County who sent her a box of select ladies' clothing."[7]

She was adored by the foot soldiers. "Much of her confidence came from the unabashed adoration of the common soldiers. If she missed the attentions of a husband or the fulfillment of her romantic dreams, she now claimed a thousand ardent loves who exalted her name or shyly brought her gifts of nosegays and apples. Officers saluted her and a steady stream of young fellows in blue made their way toward her door on Seventh street. They came to thank her, to show her their improvement in health, or to chat about the battles they had been through together. The man from the doorway of the Lacy House, whose leg Clara had bound in a life-saving tourniquet, called one afternoon. To her surprise, he dispensed with traditional greetings, blurting out instead, "You saved my life." . . . she received an invitation to visit the men in Ward 17 of Lincoln Hospital. Each man had been wounded at Fredericksburg and treated at the Lacy House before being brought to the capital city. As she entered the room they shouted and applauded, some poor fellows falling back in their beds from the effort. She would not exchange the memory of their three great cheers, Barton later admitted, 'for the wildest hurrahs that ever greeted the ear of conqueror or king.' "[8]

1. Historian R. H. Bremer. Source unknown.
2. *Clara Barton: Professional Angel*, by Elizabeth Brown Pryor, University of Pennsylvania Press, Copyright 1987, ISBN 0-8122-8060-1, p. 89.
3. Ibid., p. 97.
4. Ibid., p. 99.
5. Ibid., p. 61.
6. Ibid., p. 62.
7. Ibid., p. 108.
8. Ibid., p. 109

The above quoted with special arrangement with the University of Pennsylvania Press.

THE RED CROSS YEARS

Because of her experiences in our own Civil War, when Russia and Turkey were at war in 1877, Clara Barton saw the needs and "hit upon the idea of forming an American Red Cross Society which would collect contributions for the sufferers in Turkey and Russia."[1]

She contacted the International Red Cross Committee in Geneva and was authorized to proceed with an American Red Cross. Then she did much lobbying for several months, needing the strength she had gradually been regaining after another five year period of illness and forced inactivity. The whole problem was that the United States needed to ratify the Geneva Convention, which had initiated the International Red Cross, so one could be started in this country. Yet Congress was reluctant to do so. Eventually a joint Senate/House resolution was passed to "make formal and official of the Geneva Convention as asked by Miss Clara Barton."[2]

But it died in committee. Clara continued to publicize the potential group and eagerly awaited a new president. Garfield heard her proposal and requested the new Secretary of State, James G. Blaine, to hear her story. Then the Secretary of War, Robert Lincoln, and Secretary of the Treasury, Robert Windham, both promised support. On May 21, 1881, a small group met to adopt a constitution of the American Association of the Red Cross; the group was in existence and Barton was elected its first president.

To understand the whole woman, a reader should know the following event, which the author enters here as interesting extranea.

Her public life came to a screaming halt when she was ousted as head of the American Red Cross. George Elsey, President Emeritus of the ARC, says she was forced-out in disgrace.

The ARC was apparently in good health with Clara Barton having single-handedly founded and nurtured it for a quarter of a century, but trouble was brewing. Some of the directors were dissatisfied and infighting had developed. While Clara was in Russia on business, Mount Pelee had erupted, killing 40,000 people on Martinique. Clara blamed the ARC board for not sending a relief force. She had relied on them to act and their failure to do so created great disenchantment.

Then she learned of a plan to replace her at the ARC December 1902 meeting and decided to act on her own. "She prepared some sweeping provisions, giving the president the right of appointment over virtually every committee, abolishing the Board of Directors, and essentially, eliminating any controlling power from the Executive Committee. Of course this created a furor at the December 9 meeting (but) by a narrow margin the revised bylaws were approved . . . To cap this triumph Barton was elected president for life."[3]

Mabel Boardman, who had been a leader of the opposition,

"considered the techniques Barton had used to be dishonorable and probably illegal. (She and others) now had proof that (Clara) meant to rule the ARC in any way she could. Late in December they wrote to President Theodore Roosevelt who, like all his predecessors, had the honorary position as chairman of the ARC Board of Advisors. They complained of Barton's highhanded tactics at the board meeting and shared their worry that the new bylaws did not contain enough safeguards against absolute rule by Barton or any other president."[4]

"A few days after the new year, (Roosevelt) moved to sever all official ties his administration held with the American Red Cross . . . In the letter (the President) accused her of 'loose and improper' financial arrangements and censored the 'very irregular and arbitrary proceedings' at the meeting on December 9. He requested that his name and the names of his cabinet officers, be removed from the Red Cross board of advisors, and he hinted that the official connection between the organization and the American government had been completely broken."[5]

Boardman and others delved deeply into Barton's personal and financial life and not too long thereafter forced her to resign. Clara was 81 years old. Boardman took control and retained it until 1946.

After the Red Cross aided victims of the Johnstown, Pennsylvania flood in 1889, Clara had a temporary shelter in that area taken down and the lumber stored in Washington for future use. Within two years it was used to construct a building at Glen Echo, Maryland, to be the offices of the American Red Cross and also Clara's personal living quarters after 1897. Today it is the Clara Barton National Historic Site, being managed by the National Park Service.

Clara reached the end of her years and died April 12, 1912, at Glen Echo, leaving behind a lifetime of humanitarian work, a great contribution to the world, a strong woman who had accomplished much more than she ever admitted to herself.

The reader should obtain a copy of Elizabeth Pryor's book, footnoted herein and consider it for further reading. It is a masterful effort and well deserves attention.

1. *Clara Barton: Professional Angel*, by Elizabeth Brown Pryor, University of Pennsylvania Press, copyright 1987, ISBN 0-8122-8060-1, p. 188.
2. Ibid., p. 195.

3. Ibid., p. 338.
4. Ibid., p. 339.
5. Ibid., p. 62.

The above material quoted by special arrangement with the University of Pennsylvania Press.

AN ERRATIC EGO

Clarissa Harlowe Barton is another great leader in the history of nursing. The Angel of the Battlefield, named so for her work on American battlefields during our Civil War, may be the antithesis of today's nurse. The modern nurse has been taught to honor and respect Clara Barton, just as many of us were taught in grade school. But Clara was a woman driven to service more for a need for recognition and self-justification than by pure selfless service. Today's nurse is more apt to be less self-centered and hopeful of alleviating pain, promoting healing and being of service to her patients—for their betterment, not for her personal recognition.

But before we seem too bitter toward poor Clara, let's picture her home in North Oxford, Massachusetts. Born on Christmas day 1821, she was one of five siblings, the others all being at least ten years her senior. Her father was a strong-willed, quick-tempered man who went into fits of rages. Her mother was so conservative that she saved everything, even keeping pies in the basement rather than destroying them when they were dangerously old. Clara's sister Dolly, had to be kept locked up at home in a room with barred windows after she went insane when Clara was six. In this family came a shy, timid child, an excellent student, even brilliant.

Is it any wonder that young Clara spent her life wondering what she was, where she belonged and once said that she could remember nothing about her childhood but fear?

All during her life Clara was affected by those people. She nursed people in the community, she nursed a brother for two years, she proved to be a loving person, but she never was free of worry of potential insanity. No matter how much she served on the Civil War battlefields, no matter how well she taught school children, she always strove to receive the recognition she never once had at home.

15

It drove her to such secretiveness about herself that she could not share the personal aspects of her life.

Much of this came to the surface in fairly recent years when her personal diaries of 50 years were discovered bricked up behind a wall in her Glen Echo, Maryland home and office of the American Red Cross, during a restoration. As curator of that Clara Barton House, Elizabeth Brown Pryor used these diaries as prime reference material to author *Clara Barton, Professional Angel*, copyright in 1987. She had previously published *Clara Barton National Historic Site.*[1]

"Besides Clara's own voluminous correspondence, author Pryor used letters and reminiscences of lovers, a grandniece who probed her aunt's venerable facade, and doctors who treated her nervous disorders."

She spent much of her life "patching up the lives of those around her when her own was rent and frayed."[2]

"She became so concerned that she wasn't contributing to her family (that) she "found purpose in caring for her sister Sally's children . . . she befriended many of North Oxford's poorer families . . . During a smallpox epidemic that occurred in her early teens, she . . . nursed several families until she herself came down with the disease. . . In one instance she carried a lantern and led the way out in the midnight darkness while Mr. Clemence carried the casket of one of his children and buried it."[3]

"There seemed to be a weak link that prevented her attaining personal happiness. What is found . . . is a personality often at odds with itself . . . a merciless, driving force, a shattering insecurity, a demanding and erratic ego. When she wrote that her work had been accomplished 'against fearful odds' she was speaking of the many battles waged internally, the long fight against crippling depression and fear of insanity that grew out of her need to excel and her belief that she had never done enough to secure a place in the world."[4]

At age 18 she began teaching and was very successful. There is even one episode when she was given such an unruly class that she used a riding whip on one boy and thus subdued the entire group. Even at age 29 she went to the Clinton, New York Liberal Institute; she wanted education and was ahead of her time. Her mother died in 1851 and Clara returned home, finding no need for her there, went to visit friends in Hightstown, New Jersey. She was bored, went back into teaching and started her own free school in Bordon-town, New Jersey, because she felt sorry for children of poor parents who couldn't afford the private subscription schools. It became a successful public school. But Clara was still lost and went to Washington, D.C. at age 33 to become an officer worker in the Patent Office. Actually, she was the only female employed by the U.S. Government at the time.[4] "In reality, her whole life had been spent in a search of the public acclaim that served as a salve for the indifference of her family."[5]

In later years she dyed her hair and lied about it . . . "she cosmetically lowered her age when the press inquired or the census taker came round. Her obsession with obscuring even the smallest details of her life reflected a sad lack of self-esteem and a need to project an image of perfection."[5]

1. *Clara Barton: Professional Angel*, by Elizabeth Brown Pryor, University of Pennsylvania Press, Copyright, 1987. ISBN 0-8122-8060-1, p. 109.

2. Ibid. Book's jacket.

3. Ibid., p. 17. Pryor quoting "Honora Connors to Clara Barton, February 15, 1987 — apparently a letter.

4. "Clara Barton," Produced by the Division of Publications, National Park Service, U.S. Department of the Interior, Washington, D.C., 1981. Handbook #110 of the National Park Handbook Series.

5. Pryor, pp. x and 14.

The above material quoted by special arrangement with the University of Pennsylvania Press.

YOO HOO, DOCTOR BLUE, I NEED YOU

The other day we received three heart attack victims, each brought into our emergency room while I was on duty. Due to the excellent Doctor Blue team available, all three lives were saved. But I wonder if the families of these victims fully appreciated what had happened.

My respect for Doctor Blue teams is beyond imagination because they keep us alive many times — and specially trained nurses are right in there prominently as part of the team.

Whenever I see a person, usually a man of my own vintage, being fought over so efficiently by a Red Room Cardiac Team, trying to keep that person alive, I want to get on a pedestal and orate.

Why? Because I want the world to see the pattern of that physical body. I want the world to see that huge, bulbous stomach that is invariably present. I want to force the world to see what fat has probably done.

Here on this gurney almost always there is a small head and shoulders, tapering legs and feet, with an intervening mountain in between. Here is thirty to fifty pounds of excess weight trying to kill this dear soul who has refused to give up the beer, the liquor, the French fries, the heavy food, until a precipitated heart attack knocks him flat.

I want him to see the Doctor Blue teams run furiously to the Red Rooms to try to save his life. I want him to see the intensity of physicians, nurses, other specialists, fight to keep him alive. I want to motivate him (or her, of course) to trim away some of that weight and to give his heart a chance.

I'd like to give every overweight person a couple of 20 pound sacks of salt or flour and say "Friend, this is what you are carrying around *as an extra* and using to kill yourself."

I'd like to tell him to ask a member of the healthcare team how to get that weight under control.

WAR ZONE

My hospital resides smack in the middle of a decrepit, drug-infested neighborhood. Shells of empty houses line the littered streets. Businesses are gone, except for the ever-popular corner bar and the omnipresent dealers. By day, the sidewalks are deserted, except for a handful of children. Two little girls sit on a stained mattress and play with armless Barbie dolls. A group of young boys play with objects scavenged from some littered, vacant lot, while their moms stare aimlessly from doorways. At nght, the activity picks up. As I wind my way to work, I am often treated to the sight of emaciated, dirty women flinging their shirts over their bare breasts to advertise their availability. Dealers peek into my car, stopped at a red light, and display their wares.

I don't know why I continue to work here. I guess it's because if I don't, nobody else will. This place is where my family once called home. My grandfather worked at the old wicker warehouse, long burned down. My grandmother once roller skated on these same streets that now spark with broken crack vials. My dad hit his first homerun over in that playground. At least I think that is the playground. Now it is only a bunch of weeds choking the rested skeleton of a swing set.

Here's the hospital. Like the neighborhod, it obviously has seen better days. The ICU is a hybrid between *2001* and *MASH*. In the seventies the former one-room ward had been hastily partitioned to give the illusion of private rooms. A curtain serves as a doorway. Next to the manual crank-beds are relatively recent cardiac monitors. Unfortunately, the unit was supposed to be renovated and modernized last year, but the hospital declared bankruptcy instead. Now the unit is a cluttered hodge-podge of old and new.

This particular 7 P.M.-7 A.M. shift promises to be a busy one. It's Friday night and that in itself brings trouble. The phone rings, and I am given report on my new admission: a 32 year-old known drug abuser in respiratory arrest. It seems that this fine, upstanding, citizen arrived in the ER barely breathing. The girl friend, staggering and obviously high herself, informed the nurse that "Jim" had ingested a week's worth of Valium and an unknown amount of Xanax and had then finished his spree with some speedballs (a mixture of heroin and cocaine injected into the veins). Jim was intubated, connected to a ventilator, and a tube passed into his stomach to remove whatever else was left down there. An arterial line was inserted to monitor his blood pressure, and to remove blood samples without sticking him, his veins being practically nonexistent from his drug abuse. The EKG and blood tests revealed cardiac muscle damage, so Jim was started on IV nitroglycerine to reduce further damage. Because the nitroglycerine, as well as the multitude of drugs he'd already ingested, was lowering his blood pressure, the ER doctor ordered IV Dopamine. In addition to raising the blood pressure, Dopamine also increases the blood flow to the vital organs of the body.

In this state Jim arrives at my unit. I hook up the various lines to the bedside monitor and suck accumulated secretions out of his endotracheal tube, and proceed to finish my assessment of the man. During this time the doctors whirl around the room, examining the numbers on the screen and shouting: "His pressure is dropping! Jack up the dopamine. How many mikes (micrograms) is he getting now? Okay, that's good. I want his systolic above 90. Call me with any problems."

I notice Jim's eyelids beginning to flutter.

"Oh, Mike! Before you leave the unit, can I get a verbal order for some Pavulon?" Pavulon is a muscle-paralyzing drug. I knew that Jim was probably going to be quite combative when he finally awoke and I had no desire to spend the rest of my shift wrestling with him.

"Um, I don't think that's a good idea right now. The girl friend wasn't sure about all the types or amounts of drugs he ingested and I want to keep the amount we give him to a minimum. Just keep him restrained and do your best." Mike shrugs and leaves the unit. I check on my other patient, who is stable and ready to be moved to the floor, then return to Jim.

The next few hours flew by. Admission paperwork is a royal pain in the butt, but necessary. As the lawyers say "If it wasn't written it wasn't done." Doctors are not the only ones who can be sued today. Unless I chart everything, I cannot prove that I performed the

actions, should I be sued. Some patients sue the hospital, figuring
that the hospital's insurance coverage will pay for the damages, and
no one gets hurt. What a myth! What they don't know is that the
same hospital can turn around and sue the nurse for damages!

A noise brings me back to Jim's room. He has managed to loosen
one of the restraints and is attempting to remove the endotracheal
tube. His eyes are wide with terror. I try to shorten the restraints but
I'm too late. The tube is out and Jim gasps for breath.

"Call anesthesia, STAT!"

In an instant everyone is in the room. Both the anesthesiologist
and Mike decide that Jim can breathe on his own with supplemental
oxygen. Jim is definitely getting better. Each attempt at pulling out
his lines is stronger than the previous one. Slowly, I wean off the
Dopamine to compensate for his renewed vigor. The drugs are finally leaving his system.

My twelve-hour shift is half over. I am exhausted, but Jim isn't.
His shouts bring me and my coworkers into the toom.

"Get me the fuck out of here now. I want out! You hear me? I'm
leaving! You can't keep me in here!" Everything at maximum
volume.

He is sitting straight up in bed, oxygen mask pulled up onto his
head.

While the other nurses try to calm him down, I run to the phone
and summon the house doctor.

"Mike, he's freaking out. I have the leather restraints ready. Any
suggestions?"

"I'll be right up," Mike replies.

Jim is now swinging at the othe rnurses and has one leg over the
side rail. I try to reason with him.

"Jim, you are still very sick. You are in the hospital, in the Intensive Care Unit. I am your nurse, Rita." Jim has now stopped moving
and is looking at me very intently. I continue.

"You almost died last night. If you leave now you may not make
it home. You need to stay here and get better. Please put your leg
back into bed . . . "

"Go fuck yourself, bitch" he yells. Mike enters the room and attempts to reason with the man, only to be subjected to an even
uglier diatribe than mine.

21

"Okay, pal. Forget it. If you want to go back out there and do some more drugs, fine. Let me pull out those IV lines and have you sign a form and you can leave."

Jim looks satisfied and Mike leaves the room. Jim has us in a tight spot. Although we believe he needs to stay here, he is considered competent under the law and we cannot force him to receive treatment. With an unconscious person, consent is implied but that description no longer fits Jim.

Mike returns with a form know as "Against Medical Advice." This form states that the patient willingly is leaving the hospital and refusing treatment even though the physician and hospital staff have informed the patient that it is not in his best interests to do so. The entire hospital is relieved from liability should the patient experience any harm from this decision to leave prematurely. Jim eagerly signs the form and Mike and I remove the remaining IV lines. I hand Jim his clothes and he slowly dresses himself. His heart, although considerably weakened from the ordeal, is functioning enough for him to feel cured. He wants that next fix and wants it badly enough to leave the hospital and to kill himself by degrees. Now dressed, he stumbles out to the visitor's lounge to call his girlfriend.

The horizon is turning pink. My shift is nearly over. The day shift is filtering in and activity in the unit starts accelerating. All of this is lost on me. I am thoroughly disgusted and angry.

"I break my back and keep that idiot alive" I think, "and the son of a bitch signs out AMA (Against Medical Advice)! After all the expense of effort, energy and personnel! Not to mention medications and equipment. We save his life and he up and staggers out the front door."

A coworker, after hearing about my night, attempts to console me.

"Don't worry," she says, "this happens all the time. There was nothing you could have done. They come in here barely breathing, we revive them, and they go out and do it all over again. You would think they'd learn, but they don't. He'll be back."

As I drive home I look for Jim on the corners and in the shadows of the soul-less buildings. I think I seem him in every face along the street. When I arrive home, I glance at the morning paper, wondering if he is still alive.

So much for the War on Drugs.

Rita Jablonski, RN
Philadelphia, PA

Postscript: I apologize about the language used herein and realize it is a bit strong. On the other hand, I deal with this type of thing on a daily basis and think the language conveys the feeling and flavor of the incident. People tend to gloss over the daily challenges that nurses meet and idealize our work. But the reality of the situation is that nurses tolerate a great deal of abuse, usually at the hands of people like Jim. People need to be aware of what some of us face on a daily basis. This is not an isolated case. (RJ)

TWO VERY SPECIAL PATIENTS

I started my nurse's training in Rochester, Minnesota, in February, 1938, at St. Mary's hospital. I well remember the original Doctors Will and Charlie Mayo, and the son, and a Doctor Coventry who was from Duluth, all outstanding physicians, as the world knows. We had Doctor Will and Doctor Charlie on orientation.

Swimming was a required activity but I always had severe headaches after swimming so my instructor insisted I go to the clinic to be examined. It was suggested I go home, so I did, to Illinois. Soon I went to Kankakee where I was interviewed by the same order of nurses I finally joined. I had also heard of a fine hospital in Champagne-Urbana, to which I wrote telling them of my training at St. Mary's. I was accepted for classes there starting September 8, 1938. I spent three years there and was capped in 1941.

Now I'm looking forward to September, 1991, when I'll observe my fiftieth year as a practicing registered nurse. I want that one more year and hope my health holds up.

There were twelve of us who finished that class together. Today, in 1990, all are still alive.

I agree with Dorothy, whose story appears elsewhere in this book, that we had seven to eight hours of supervision daily, all week long. I've seen the girls in the St. Petersburg Tampa area, for example, come on in the morning and two girls have one patient between them. We used to give at least two baths every morning.

Yes, we had good training and were quickly offered supervisory positions.

I had my daughter in April, the year after I was graduated. During five months of this time I also cared for a lady living on a farm adjoining ours, in Illinois. When we had to hospitalize her in Kankakee, the hospital authorities came to me and offered me the night supervisor job. This was quite a compliment to me as such a young nurse, and I accepted. I realized my lack of training in emergency room could be a problem and I was determined to learn ER nursing. So I started working doing private duty and whenever a patient was brought into ER I was called down to observe and to learn. Previously I didn't even know where supplies were kept in ER.

Just two years ago I took care of a thirty-one year old AIDS patient. I kept avoiding that contact because AIDS was such a new disease and we didn't know much about it. Finally, I was ready for an AIDS patient.

Pete was a very nice gentleman, who needed nursing partly to provide scheduled medication. He had overdosed on medication by being confused over dosages and time.

He was such a good man. A very few of the nurses were unkind to him but I insisted we not make judgments. That's right. You'd never know he was an AIDS patient because he looked as well as you or I.

I got to know Pete unusually well. Once he said "I resent the way some of the nurses treat me," to which I replied "I can understand that, Pete, but you must remember this is a new area and we're all trying to learn more about this disease." We talked, long, long hours.

Pete did much for the hospital community. He was somewhat like a nurse's aide, volunteering in many ways. I got to know him very well in the eight or nine months I cared for him. He was so open with me that he'd tell me all events that happened to him while he lived in California. The first indication that he had AIDS was when a sarcoma appeared on an extremity.

What a weight for him to bear.

I've just finished reading a book called "AIDS-The Caregiver's

Handbook," which is excellent. Good for anyone caring for or working around AIDS patients. I strongly recommend it.

The full identification is: "AIDS-The Caregiver's Handbook," by Ted Eidsen, New York, St. Martin's Press, 1988. Identified as ISBN # 0-312-02151-6.

Many people don't realize that AIDS is not easy to catch. Of course, if you have a cut or a wound, no matter how small, you could get infected. Caregivers of such patients are strongly urged to wash their hands very frequently.

Pete had two roommates who were both gay. You'd never have known it by appearances, but Pete told me they were.

My heart just went out when Pete died. He had gone out one day and had something alcoholic to drink, which is a big no-no for AIDS victims. When he came home, he lay down on the couch for a brief time. When one of the roommates came home, he gave Pete a Darvocet (which had been prescribed for him) for Pete's headache. Later on the roommate checked him and found he had died.

You should have seen Pete's house. That man was very talented. He liked to cook, loved art, and was very sensitive to other people's needs.

I'm only glad that he didn't go through a long, painful dying process and I'm very pleased that I was there when he needed someone like me.

I also took care of David, an eighteen-year old paraplegic. He had been in the service in California, was riding a motorcycle, stopped in a lane of vehicles at a semaphore, when the truck in front of him rammed backwards into him, causing the loss of all four limbs and his ability to talk.

After his treatment in California, they transported him to his parent's home in Florida.

I was taking care of David in the nursing home where I worked at that time and got to know his mother. David hadn't been in that home very long but he knew which people liked him and which ones didn't. Because he couldn't talk, some people stupidly thought he couldn't think.

He was being tube fed and I was determined that we'd teach him how to eat properly, at least to chew and to swallow. So I worked laboriously with him toward that goal. Gradually he made progress and could swallow when I told him to do so. I soon had that tube out of his throat.

I used to sit and read to David quite a lot. Some of the girls resented that, stating I was wasting my time. "But," I said, "that's my job. I can't sit and do nothing. I want to help him."

I suggested to the physicians that we bring in a speech therapist and they did. It was interesting to watch them work as a team.

Some afternoons I'd take David outside in his chair, to get the warm sun. No one else would do that though.

The mother eventually insisted that David be entered into a VA hospital. The first week he was there I visited him and found they were having problems with him. David would simply do nothing for them. They were using a different approach than I had used, so they let me feed him. They saw how well it worked and were very pleased I had come by. It was a good experience for all of us.

It's amazing to think that David could help others, but he found ways to do it in spite of being a paraplegic, in spite of being so helpless that he had to be lifted in and out of bed. What a strong will he had.

I learned that he liked music so one day brought him a Bill Cosby record. You know how delightfully interesting Cosby can be. I was at the desk one day when David was listening to Cosby and another nurse said "What's that strange noise?" It was David, laughing. I don't think any of us had ever heard him laugh before. He was learning to do things that any normal person could do — but that's something he would never be — normal, that is.

Although I'm in good health for a nurse about to observe her fiftieth year of service, I've had my problems too and have cause to appreciate good nursing.

When we lived in North Carolina I was returning to a house from which we'd just moved, intending to clean it. I went off the road in a mountainous area, driving a little GMC truck. I went down the mountainside 160 feet, struck a big boulder and flipped six or seven times. It was one of those weird exceptions to the rule — when I was lucky *not* to be wearing a seat belt.

Richard, my son, went down later to look at the wreck and the roof of the cab w as pushed down flat. If I'd been stationary, belted, I'd have been crushed as flat as a pancake.

All the windows were shattered, so they pulled me out the rear window. I could tell the emergency people my name but that was all. I had a broken pelvis, one broken rib on the left side, five or six on the right side, a punctured lung, cuts on the face and a big bump on the head.

The children had wanted to go with me but Richard had said no. Had they been in the cab or in the truck body, they undoubtedly would have been killed.

I was lucky just to be alive and have thanked God many times for that, and I was grateful to have good nurses to help me recover.

Sometime I'll tell you about my experiences in Japan.

Marjorie J. Lowrey, RN
Marathon, Florida

HOW PANTSUITS CAME TO OUR HOSPITAL

It's hard to believe that it happened so long ago. Now I no longer wear white but blue scrubs and they are furnished by the hospital. So we have come a long way.

I remember when I started nurse's training, as it was called, in the early fifties. The uniforms were almost to our ankles and they were all cotton, starched so stiffly they could stand by themselves. But the hospital did our uniforms, so it was no big labor on our part.

However, when we walked down the halls or into a patient's room the skirt made quite a noise—swish, swish, crackle, crackle.

The caps were just as stiff and every school of nursing had a particular style, so you could tell where a nurse was trained by looking at her cap. Why were we so proud of our caps? Well, there was the first six months of training, called "probation" and we student nurses were called "probies." If we survived the probation period, and many did not, we had a big ceremony and were capped. A bareheaded nurse was immediately recognized as one with little experience or knowledge.

Just as other styles change, so did the uniform and cap. Women started wearing nylon and polyester—no more starch. Dresses became shorter. Women stopped wearing hats.

Just think back a few generations. Women wore veils and hats.

Perhaps because they only washed their hair once a week or, perhaps in Florence Nightingale's day, a lot of people had lice.

We wanted to wear the same type of clothes that women were wearing outside the hospital. We felt more comfortable in slacks. So we took a survey and found that our hospital was the only one in our city that did not allow pantsuits. So we passed around a petition requesting that the dress code be changed so we could dress as nurses did elsewhere. We were tired of buying uniforms which were so short you could see the nurse's underwear when she bent over. The doctors said they didn't want the nurses to change; they enjoyed seeing the legs. So then we were really determined to wear pantsuits.

Our petition was ignored by nursing administration. I don't remember the exact year but it was between 1975 and 1978, so we decided we needed a test case.

I was working the night shift—11 P.M. to 7 A.M. One night when I was the only nurse scheduled to work in ER (the emergency room) I wore my new pantsuit. It had a tunic style top that came down below the hips, almost as long as some of the dresses nurses were wearing.

The evening supervisor saw me as I came to work and said "Has the dress code been changed?" I replied "I haven't heard a thing since the petition was signed several months ago."

She reported my uniform to the night supervisor, who called my head nurse, who called her supervisor, who called the Director of Nursing.

By this time it was after midnight and all the evening shift nurses had gone home.

So, my head nurse's supervisor called me and said "I hear you are wearing a pantsuit" and I replied "Yes, I am."

She said "You'll have to go home and change." I replied "I live quite a ways and I might not get back for a long time." To which she said "You'll just have to remove the pants."

So I did, wearing a white lab coat over my long tunic top and white panty hose.

The next morning the head nurse and supervisor were there bright and early to decide what punishment I should receive for such insubordinate behavior. Would it be dismissal? Three days without pay? Written reprimand that would be part of my permanent record?

I went home feeling quite upset. Then I started getting phone calls. Other nurses told me if any punitive action were taken by the administration they would have a massive sick call throughout the hospital.

In a few days I was told the administration had decided that a verbal reprimand was all that I would receive. Shortly after that we received notice that we could wear pantsuits. Of course certain supervisors were required to wear dresses for years.

So that's the way uniform pants came to our big hospital — which was not in the town where I now live.

Clarissa Rownd, RN
Fountain Hills, Arizona

THE EVOLUTION OF A VOICE

I attended Augsburg college after high school and was a future voice major. Within a year I knew that I would rather dissect a frog than a piece of music. Nursing had been of interest to me at times throughout my childhood and Dr. Erwin Mickelberg, a professor of anatomy and physiology at Augsburg, encouraged me to think about attending Deaconess school of nursing in Minneapolis. Little did I know that I would still be a voice major . . . in a different way.

I was accepted into the program and in the fall of 1974 was capped as a Deaconess student. Approximately one and a half years into the three-year program, wedding bells rang and my new husband's job took us to rural Iowa. I was eight months pregnant with our second daughter when I entered the ADN (two-year Associate Degree in Nursing program) at Iowa central community college in Fort Dodge, Iowa, and was graduated in July, 1979; I was three months pregnant with our wonderful third daughter by then.

My first jobs as a registered nurse were in rural communities with 20-35 bed hospitals. Rural nursing is uniquely different from specialty nursing. I considered myself to be jack-of-all-trades and master of none. The jobs were challenging and demanded flexibility.

There was tremendous stress. The role required diverse job performance—assisting with the birth of a healthy baby within minutes of giving comfort to a grieving family who had just watched their loved one die. In a way, one event balanced out the other, but the questioning began. What would life be like beyond nursing? Is this where I belong?

As a rural nurse I took care of whatever walked in the doors—assessment skills assisted me to survive. I didn't know how significant and valuable my nursing was to patient care because many patients, at that time, credited physicians only for successes related to their health care. The reality was that a lot of situations required quick nursing decisions and even medical treatments (covered by standing orders) without the presence of a physician. I, as a nurse, made a difference to people's lives without a physician but the system made sure I didn't get credit for my actions. I knew something was wrong—something felt out of balance.

I remember one night spending five of nine hours in an emergency room with the same physician. The night was horrible. The physician intimidated me repeatedly in front of the patients. At first I didn't say anything and, as the night progressed, the abusive treatment continued; I felt angry and teary. At the end of the night I pulled the physician aside and said to him "This has been a hell of a night for you and a hell of a night for me." That conversation was the starting point for one of the most effective behaviors I have learned as a nurse—*direct communication*—and I had a voice, but it was a while before I recognized the evolving voice was different from the singing voice I knew.

After nearly six years of rural nursing in Iowa and then Kansas, my husband's job brought us to a town near Lincoln, Nebraska. I was discouraged with nursing. The work was exhausting—demanding patients, crazy hours, no decision-making power and low pay. None the less, I applied for an intensive care/coronary care position at St. Elizabeth's in Lincoln.

Within six months I knew I had made the right decision to continue questioning my role as a nurse. Before a year had passed I was committed to nursing. What made the difference? Basically it was the environment in which I practiced nursing. I had a nurse manager who said "You are the one doing patient care. What can I do to make sure you can do that?" She wasn't telling me how to be a nurse; she was there to create the environment in which I could perform well and be recognized for my contributions to patient care. I looked for professional role models in the work place and found them—Joyce, Lynette and Susan. I though WHEE—a breath of fresh air. Maybe I could begin to love nursing again, begin to discover my voice.

I began to evaluate my role in the system, the inbalances I had felt before now taking on new perspectives. Education made a trememdous difference in the ICU/CCU and I not only became committed to nursing, but looked forward to finding an opportunity to return to academia for a BSN (Bachelor of Science in Nursing). A move to Minnesota allowed me to realize the dream and in June, 1990 I was graduated with distinction from the University of Minnesota.

As I reflect on how I made a difference in peoples' lives there are several experiences that stay with me. One was with an elderly lady, Louise, in Kansas. She was admitted to a three bed intensive care unit, in one of the rural hospitals, with chest pain. A heart attack was ruled out but more tests concluded that she had metastatic cancer. Chemotherapy was tried unsuccessfully. At the time, one of the nursing interventions I used to assist my patient to deal with the emotions related to illness was music. I would bring my guitar to work and sing a favorite song. I did this for Louise. She and her husband, Jim, cried as I sang the song they had chosen, "In the Garden." Before long they were talking about memories and laughing about some of the experiences they'd had in their lives. We discovered through conversation that they lived in the same community as I and I was invited to their home.

Unbeknownst to me I was introduced to my first nursing experience in public health/home health. I was able to see Louise in her home environment, amongst the numerous paintings she had done. I watched her create homemade cards and realized that the artist had a need to be remembered, so on Mother's day I sang a song that I had written for her entitled "The Artist." She became teary, not because she was dying, but because she would be remembered.

A man patient sent me several letters after he left the hospital.

31

NURSE

He had lived on the prairies for most of his life and had a need to maintain the independence he valued. I was able to hear his concern about his own illness through conversation. He said to me, after I sang a couple of songs, "I paint pictures and even write some poetry." I asked him to share one of his poems and this is what he said:

> This little shack on the prairie
> Is home sweet home to me
> The sow belly, beans and coffee
> Are always calling me.
> On a very cold night in the winter
> With all wild creatures in bed
> I throw cow chips on the heater
> And throw blankets over my head.
> I dream of before I homesteaded
> Of my youth, far, far away
> And all the joys of pure living
> When all the kids came to play.
> But now here on the prairie
> I'm a man, no longer a kid
> I wouldn't trade all of my troubles
> For the joy a rich man has.
> My shack is dirty
> My shirts are torn
> My pants are out at the knees
> I don't worry for what I can't help
> I live as I darned well please.
>
> Harold Pickens

I heard Harold saying that he valued what he had on the prairies and institutional living wouldn't necessarily be his cup of tea. I put his poem to music and sang it for him, and he has given me permission to quote the poem and to tell his story. How wonderful to hear that he made it home. He wrote in one of his letters, "It's so nice to know that you cared about me."

I don't believe it was words but my singing voice alone that made a difference in the experiences. The stories reveal the voice of nursing that I had not recognized earlier in my career—a caring voice, the heart of today's healthcare system.

My statement will be and should be talent. The author of this book, William Hull, said that he had heard that nursing had lost its professionalism because of higher pay rates. One cannot deny that there are nurses who are there as a means to an end, nurses who are bitter and angry because of use and abuse by the healthcare system. They decide to stay in the system and are a reactive voice; in some ways they keep the system honest. Looking back on where I've been, I can understand where the reactive behaviors are coming from. They demand salaries that reflect the work being done and are the ones who say "No more money for equipment and technology. Put the money in your nurses."

A new type of nurse is evolving—one who chooses a pro-active voice and paints a different picture of nursing. They agree that nurses are worth higher salaries, but seek to prove worth by other means. These nurses are beginning to do research and data collection in the practice environment and are proposing cost-efficient ways of delivering quality patient care thereby making their worth known to the healthcare community.

There are also nurses who are neither reactive nor proactive in the profession who watch their peers for direction and are there because they hear the same voice most nurses have heard at one time or another.

As I continued to grow in nursing, I began to understand where nursing's future is in the health care system. I speak not only of hospital nurses but of public health nurses, school nurses, nurse practitioners, nurse clinicians, nurse educators, researchers, etc. Opportunities need to continue for one-to-one caring, but nurses will not always be able to do the caring on a one-to-one basis. The current health care environment requires that nurses be creative about caring. Nursing resources are limited and utilized extensively in a high tech environment. Questions such as: What are the resources the patient has to meet health care needs? Family? Pastors? Friends? Someone to sit in the room when the nights get long and lonely, someone to listen when emotions are overwhelming. How can the nurse create an environment where caring is central?

I have evolved into a nurse who knows her singing and her caring voice and I seek future opportunities to be a pro-active voice for nursing. Administrators, physicians, and professional organizations must create an environment wherein nurses can define and control their practice so that the heart stays in the health care system of tomorrow.

Nursing makes a difference!

M. J. Swanson, RN BSN
Elk River, Minnesota

---

42 YEARS OF NURSING

The three year course I took—we went 36 months, not nine months for three years—had classes the year around; we worked eight to ten hours in training, plus two to four hours in classes. The first year we had two weeks off at Christmas time and then we went two and a half years without a day off. So you can see we received a lot of training. On Sundays we only worked six hours.

At the end of six months we were assigned a full load at eight hours. I believe we were getting better academic instruction and probably able to give better bedside care than today's nurses. We were at the end of an era, after which instructional methods changed. I highly esteem today's nurses but sometimes wish they had the rigors of our training. For example, today's nurses put in two hours a day, three days a week, for a total of six hours of supervised training. Compare that with the eight hours which we endured every single day. With that tempo we had time to learn organizational skills which I doubt if today's nurses get a chance to learn.

As a result, we quickly went into heavy nursing responsibilities. I was a head nurse in a nearby town of 50,000 right after school. Now the girls must go through an indoctrination period and be trained in the hospital, so for the first several months they are really still in training.

They just don't have the background we had. We were very fortunate.

There were four others of my era who had the same type of training and all five of us were supervisors, because of the lengthy, detailed on-the-job training.

In my second year of nursing school I took my pediatrics—this was during the war in 1944 — and the head nurse in pediatrics asked me to be the assistant head nurse in infant pediatrics. I was an affiliated three-year nurse; although they had a few five-year nurses, they gave me the chance at the job.

A lot of my colleagues went back and got their Bachelor's degree in Science, which was necessary to be considered for these jobs. Yes, that was in a big metropolitan teaching hospital — after which I went to a big suburban trauma center. There was an awful lot of difference in these two hospitals.

In a teaching hospital I learned every day, which was very worthwhile and challenging for me. Not a day went by when I didn't learn something new.

We kept graphic charts of each patient's records. When I came on we'd get briefed for the previous 12 hours of that patient's history, thus being immediately informed about that patient. Then when the doctors came in they could grab the chart and see everything well graphed.

At Suburban we lived in nurses' quarters and sometimes they would issue a Code Orange call which means they just need nurses. So we would rush in to Intensive Care or ER, or wherever they needed us and be assigned to teams.

Of course Code Blue teams in ER and Coronary Care are for special near-death emergencies.

One time I worked in Coronary Care with another nurse, a very calm and capable person. We were both on duty one night when she said our patient, a 50 year old man, was in fibrillation and was about to die. She used the electric paddles since she was qualified as a Certified Coronary Nurse and entitled to do so. I was not. When the doctors came rushing in with the crash cart the patient was talking with the nurse, which was remarkable.

I remember one obese male patient who had legs like a kitten. He had both heart and kidney damage, a young man, probably thirty, just huge. We turned him and all of a sudden he started coding (having arrhythmias). He had so much fat we couldn't use the paddles on him at all. He was in the hospital to get rid of some of that weight.

At Downtown we had 22 bed wards, just separated by curtains. Of course in that type of hospital every patient was treated exactly equally. We had the president of a big nationally-know firm who was next to a man off the street. They would bring in these well-known business people, using other names. I remember one nurse who was caring for a patient like that when a photographer broke in and came toward him to take a photo. The nurse laid down right over him to shield and protect him from the cameraman. This was about '52 or '53. He was an old fellow and this was during the Cold War. The FBI had wanted me to keep an eye on him but I told them I had 72 patients and no way could I do that. They were interested in him because he was a registered communist.

We used to have police guards too. They'd be sitting at the foot of the bed. Sometimes the patient would get upset. One patient had a broken leg and they tied his arms and other leg to the bed. We couldn't get to him to give the proper nursing care spread-eagled like that. We asked the guard to release him because he couldn't possibly go anywhere on that badly broken leg.

It was a different life there at Downtown. Anybody who ever worked there was really dedicated. People would work beyond their shift, just to help the incoming crew turn the patients and get into their new swing. This is still true in some sections—such as my old Intensive Care Unit. Nurses are still very sincere, caring people.

You know, what goes around comes around. We had water mattresses back in 1949, but no longer because there are airbeds now. These new airbeds almost mold around a patient's body. And, of course we had those turntable beds a long time ago. The danger is in saying we know something won't work because we tried it once and it didn't work then. I know that's opinionated so I won't say that anymore.

I sure am glad I had the type of background I did. The intensive training, the work in a small 35 bed hospital in that southern Minnesota town, the experience at University Hospital during the polio outbreak and in that huge Downtown and then my last years at that excellent trauma hospital, Surburban. 42 years of nursing is a long time.

When I was in Southern Minnesota we had a lot of people coming in with malaria from being in service in the South Seas. A lot of them didn't even declare it because they wanted out. This was in the forties. They let me organize that unit, which was fun for me, because I seem to have a knack at doing that.

I was a nurse at University hospital during the polio epidemic of 1946. I had seven weeks of work without a night off. Most of those patients were adults, including a lot of pregnant women. I never had a single child polio patient. That was also about the time Sister Kenny came to the University Hospital and started her work. I think it was about 1944. I suppose you know she was called Sister Kenny in the English/Australian usage of the word "Sister" as being equivalent to "Nurse." I believe she was not a member of a Catholic order.

Patient loads have changed a lot. In the morning shifts the nurse has special problems. Patients have to go to X-Ray or Physical Therapy, or for special tests. Nurses have anywhere from five to eight patients. Five they can handle. But if they have surgical patients they require more attention. Each nurse has to plan all of the steps she must take during her shift, yet be able to adjust to interruptions and unscheduled events. Someone fails to record that your patient is due in X-Ray and you are giving them the morning bath, when the orderly or volunteer shows up to take the patient away. That has to be dealt with, so the answer is being able to adjust and to schedule.

When things started changing I went over to Downtown. In those days I'd go in, give my background and they'd say "Can you start tomorrow?" I never had to apply for a job in the old sense of the word.

Nursing experience has helped me a great deal as a mother and wife. What it did for my generation is tremendous. Just recently we had our forty-fifth nursing class reunion. Almost all of us are caretakers with a capital C. We all have emergencies in our own houses, sometimes bad ones. We seem to have the ability to look at all the alternatives, to make the decisions that have to be made. A nurse with that detailed training should have that ability because she has faced it in patient care many times. I think that's almost universal with nurses. I assume that still applies today.

I think wanting to be of service is very important. One Sunday one of the young doctors brought his daughter in and left her at the unit desk while he made his rounds. He told us "My daughter wants to be a nurse but I said to her 'Why not be a doctor'?" He thought he was being very open but everybody kind of stiffened. I said "Is there anything wrong with being a nurse?" He looked around and said "Oh, no, no." One of the nurses there belongs to Mensa and also inherited a lot of money, but she chose to be a nurse. What I'm trying to say is that nurses are still being looked down at in spite of being offered pay like seventy thousand dollars in California.

I have a special feeling for nurses. I would trust them because they are working all the time. I would trust some of them more than I would trust some doctors. They don't have the academic background of doctors but they have enough knowledcge to say 'This is wrong' and 'This is right and I am the right person to handle this situation.' Doctors are realizing the nurses' ability. Just recently I heard a doctor, leaving a nursing station, say 'Is there anything else you want from me? Do you need any orders?' Frequently the nurse gets to be part of the team, which is as it should be.

The nurse's relations with the patient's family is important too. If she has a few moments freedom from the patients she will go over and talk to the family. It's very important. Others will all pitch in to help take care of the family. That's truly a major part of patient care.

Six years ago it was starting to be that way increasingly. It isn't the big jump in salaries—but it's recognition and being part of the team that is needed. For example, this is written on Labor Day and my daughter can't find a doctor. She went to Urgent Care and they couldn't identify her problem. She thinks she has poison ivy and is about to leave for France but needs to know now. She's called her internist and can't reach him. More and more it's harder to reach specialists.

When I was at Downtown I was assigned to an elderly male patient for several months. He was such a sweet man. When he left he said "I'm going to send you some roses." I told him he didn't need to do that because I knew he was living on extremely limited funds. I said "No, that's not necessary. You can bring a card sometime if you wish" but here he came a couple of weeks later with two dozen long-stemmed red roses. Think what that meant to that man financially. I called each person who had worked with him and told them to take a rose—which was from him. We all shared in his love and remembered him for a long time.

I had a young girl patient who had cancer of the uterus. I forget the statistics but it's something like ninety-two percent recovery rate. She had surgery and came back in a few weeks and she was obviously part of the eight percent. I felt so sorry for her, thinking here I am so old and there she is, so young. She arrived with her family and boy friend. The boy friend sat there and cried until she sent him away. She told me "I have to send him away because he can't take all of this." Here she is dying and she felt sorry for him. I remember sitting down and talking with her. I told her "I'd do anything to change places with you." It's the death of the young ones that is most difficult for me.

There was another young man, about sixteen, who was walking on the street and was hit by a car. He was a quadraplegic. His mother would sit there stroking his hands and his face and he would say "Mon, I'm going to make it." Such courage touches me deeply.

Let me tell you about a funny little kid when I worked in pediatrics. He was obnoxious—no, maybe the word is precocious. He was about three. I stayed in one day to take care of him and he said to me "You have yellow teeth." Well, I do but who wants to hear it? Then I shower before work and use very expensive soap. Then he said to me "You smell." I said "Look here. We're going to be together here for the next eight hours. You quit criticizing me." It was amusing but the child needed some social skills.

But I remember joy and humor too. I was trying to remember the diagnosis of this young wife in her twenties: her husband stayed in the room with her. He slept on a cot and we let him shower in the doctors' quarters. Anyway, they didn't think she would survive. But she lived and her family threw a big bash at their lovely home, inviting everybody who had ever taken care of her. A blanket invitation—"Everybody come and spend the day." Her husband was so much in love with her it was great to see her make it. It was one of those times when you really think it was a miracle and I was glad to be part of it.

In one unit in a nursing home where I was an interim director there were three beds and a bath, plus three more beds and a bath across the nursing station. They were in a circle. One little old lady would wake up and go to the bathroom; her activity would awaken the two other little old ladies. They would wander around, then return to bed, but each would move up one bed to the next empty. When the first one came back she would crawl into the third bed, now empty. So that would go on all night, playing musical beds.

One morning the night nurse couldn't find one of the ladies—until she finally located her. She had crawled into a bed across the circle with a little old man and she was spooning him, and hugging him. A stranger, of course, but she was hugging him. This really happened.

I believe in the Living Will. I had a patient, a farmer in his late sixties, whom they brought in from a small town. He had kidney failure and faced dialysis three times a week for the rest of his life. He had not given his farm to his kids because none of them wanted to be farmers. At that time you had to have no property, no money, etc., in order to have the government pay for the dialysis. He made the decision and said "No dialysis!" Of course he didn't last long. But it's good that he had that opportunity to make the choice. This way he was able to leave some money for his wife and some for his children later on. You can't always put value on life. I think that having free choice makes a difference.

I've enjoyed my life. I'm proud to be a nurse and know I've made a contribution to a lot of people.

Dorothy Smith, RN
Minneapolis, MN

SIX WEEKS IN ICU

An 87 year old man was admitted in our hospital for trans-urethral resection procedure (TURP). Essentially there was no other medical or surgical history because he had apparently been in good health most of his life.

After just one hour in the post-operative intensive care unit (ICU) we were coding him as fibrillating, which is a "very rapid irregular contraction of the muscle fibers of the heart resulting in a lack of synchronism between heartbeat and pulse."[1]

Shock! Shock! Shock! He was given epinephrine and intubated for breathing. The works. The team stayed for an hour, first using a Swan cardiac catheter but when he went into V-tach (ventricular tachycardia, which is another type of rapid heartbeat) we employed an external pacemaker.

I've worked cardiac for three years and this code was nothing like I've seen before. There was the largest number of people I've ever seen around a patient. In ICU there are already several people in the room, prior to the Dr. Blue code. Then when the code was called more people responded and with everyone else being there my head nurse was also there handing off needed implements. She is one in a million, the reason a lot of us stay at the particular hospital.

When I looked down to start an IV on this patient, I was surprised to see concentration camp marks (tattoos) clearly distinguishable. Later, I suspected that at some point in his life he was made to be a fighter, perhaps for his own life, and perhaps it was that stamina which kept him alive this day.

Today when I walked into this man's room—he's still in ICU six weeks later—he was sitting up, brushing his own teeth, ready to take on the world. He does not flinch as I walk into his room but turns and smiles. His big brown eyes sparkle. He has one peripheral IV, a bedside monitor and other medications. He looks like he should have looked five weeks ago.

I cannot believe this 87 year old body and soul made it through what a 30 year old man may not have survived.

Now there are plans to send him home.

Mary L. Zagers, RN
Walled Lake, Michigan

HAROLD SMITHSON, MD

Harold Smithson was not "old" truly but, at age 56 the 30-year old nurses lovingly called him "Old Doctor Smithson." He was about as truly beloved as anyone could be. He had a soothing way with patients in the emergency room (ER) of the large hospital where I worked; he was gentle and kind, but also a darned good diagnostician.

If I may, I'd like to share two stories with you. The first told me by a male volunteer of many hours experience, and the second from my own witnessing.

A young boy of about nine or ten had come in to have attention given to a slash on his arm which had occurred during little league softball. He had been properly checked in and was being attended by Dr. Smithson. The doctor had given him a little local anesthesia, telling the boy that "this pin prick will sting a little." He had given the boy a few minutes time and had returned to stitch the gaping slash wound in the lad's arm.

It so happened that Dr. Smithson is very fond of baseball and, while he worked, he and the boy talked baseball, with great interest and enthusiasm. The boy, flat on his back on a gurney, was oblivious to what was happening to his arm; in fact, he couldn't see it.

As the baseball talk grew hot and heavy, the boy's attention was diverted. But, finally, he said "Doctor, aren't you going to sew up my arm or something?" To which Dr. Smithson replied "Son, I've been sewing it up. In fact, it's all done as soon as I cut off the end of this thread."

The boy was astonished. He had not realized that the good doctor had been stitching up his arm because he hadn't felt a thing.

Around this hospital we like this story as an example that such repair work can be so pain free.

My personal favorite story about the doctor occurred when we had a very obstreperous patient, a man of about 30 who was bad mouthing everybody and creating an unhappy aura in the treatment area of ER. He cursed and swore at a nurse, putting her almost in tears and making her wish she could be free of this particularly nasty patient. But she continued treating him, trying her best to relieve his pain.

As this was going on, Dr. Smithson wandered by and, caught by the patient's bad language, stopped to observe, standing back in the perimeter of the scene and saying nothing.

Suddenly the patient looked at him and said "What the hell do you want?"

To which Dr. Smithson said, "At this moment I'd like to see your rear end leaving our emergency room."

The surly patient practically yelled back at him "Well, doctor, you can just kiss my ass."

Never too easily disturbed, the good Dr. Smithson replied "Son, this is not the time to get romantic."

All the nurses and other patients and doctors within hearing broke into roaring laughter, in great appreciation of the doctor's control and wit. It only solidified his position as an outstanding and patient caregiver.

This event has gone down in history in our hospital and will long be remembered.

Dr. Smithson? He has now retired but occasionally comes back for a visit and is hailed as the returning chief. We all love him very much.

Sharon Lucas, RN
Farmington, Minnesota

A NEW HEART FOR PHIL

I have been working as a nurse in various capacities since 1973. I started as a medical-surgical nurse and helped organize the first modified intensive care unit at a large hospital. I served as assistant head nurse in that unit. After seven years, I transferred to the cardiac rehabilitation department. My ten years of experience in cardiac rehab had a profound effect on both my personal and professional life.

I always have been grateful that I selected nursing as a profession, something I wanted to do since the age of five although, aside from a far removed cousin, there are no other nurses in my family. Perhaps the fact that I was hospitalized twice before age five had some impact on my career decision. I remember one pediatric nurse who cared for me and kept in touch with my family for several years. She is no longer alive.

In 1984 I worked with Philip Jay, a man in his late thirties, the father of three young grade school children, who was recovering from a severe myocardial infarction. He also had been diagnosed as having cardiomyopathy and his prognosis was grave. In cardiac rehab our approach was holistic, addressing the body, mind, soul and spirit. As a result I found it was very easy to become close to the participants and their families. I observed Philip on several visits to our facility as an outpatient. He and his wife were struggling to hold their family together. His wife, visibly upset and emotionally distraught about his prognosis, needed much reassurance herself. My heart went out to them.

They had questions about how they were going to survive economically and, more basically, whether they had any future as a family. The doctors had told them there wasn't much they could offer him. Somehow, I felt there had to be an answer, some hope, some alternatives. It occurred to me that perhaps he would be an acceptable heart transplant candidate.

During one of his visits to the rehab center I gently pursued this option, asking him and his wife if they were familiar with this procedure. Their response to my inquiry seemed interlaced with elements of surprise and bemusement. I wonder, had my words fallen on deaf ears? After a long pause and, perhaps, taking the chance of grasping at straws, they wanted to know more. I picked up the telephone and called his cardiologist. Was there a mention of heart transplant to him in the past? The doctor suggested that that was an alternative and he would be supportive of our patient's decision should he wish to proceed.

Since heart transplants were not, at that time, performed in Nebraska, arrangements would have to be made elsewhere. Cleveland Clinic seemed the most feasible facility at that time for our candidate. Phil and Harriet were cautiously optimistic about the proposal. They were not equipped to handle the economic obligations. Where were they going to come up with the means to pay for this procedure? It seemed like a shot in the dark. I tried to be realistic yet optimistic, with comments such as "Let's have faith. Don't give up. I'll help you find a way." I contacted the head of our social services department who did the footwork and conveyed the facts to Phil's doctor, to Phil, and to me.

The next hurdle was to come up with several thousand dollars as front money. I can't remember the family's financial circumstances but money was the only obstacle at this point. We brainstormed. I contacted their priest who announced their need to the congregation. Would anyone be interested in spearheading a fundraising committee? A key person came forward. Fundraisers, including a Sweetheart Swing Valentine's Day dance, were organized. The needed money was collected. A miracle in itself, and Phil was placed on the candidate list. Since preliminary testing was required, a flight was chartered and I accompanied the couple to Cleveland. By this time Phil's condition had deteriorated and he had to lie down the entire flight. I was along to administer emergency care should the need arise.

To make a long story short, all the needed monies were collected to cover the expenses and, after a rather rocky and anxious wait, he received his heart transplant. He was the first Nebraskan to undergo this procedure. He acquired instant celebrity status and the local newspapers covered his story. He returned home feeling very blessed. It was a miracle. He still is alive and doing well. He and his wife have seen their children mature. He is a member of the heart transplant support group at the hospital and has shared his hopes and encouragements with others needing the same treatment.

Many times he has thanked me for intervening on his behalf. I feel the rewards of nursing speak for themselves in cases such as this. But then I feel nurses are like angels of mercy here on earth to serve others and to fulfill God's will. It is truly a blessing to share the joys of this glorious story with all involved. Even though I no longer work in cardiac rehab, I have to say those ten years provided some of the richest experiences I have ever had. In May 1990 I transferred to the staff development department as an instructor. I feel this is where I need to be now, but it was an emotionally ladened goodbye. I made friends with many participants.

Cec Sercl, BS, RN
Lincoln, Nebraska

IF THE HOSPITAL'S GOALS
ARE NOT MY GOALS

I believe nursing is losing a lot of its professionalism. My first instructors were very insistent that I have patience and realize that patient care must always be my primary goal. Next to that was my consideration for the family, the physician and the rest of the nursing staff. All of these, I was taught, must interact properly for the good of the patient.

Notice that I still use the word "patient" rather than "customer" or "client" because that , to me, is the very essence of nursing. I worked in home care in another state and there everyone was a client, even the physicians. At that time I did much administering of IVs in the patients' homes.

Much of the blame for the loss of professionalism must be on pay increases with the increasing attitude I see by people of all walks of life—what's in it for me. Not just hospitals, you understand.

Sixteen years ago a beginning nurse where I then worked was paid $5.70 an hour; today it is $20 there, but $11.50 is probably more average across the country. In any case, it is a necessary and deserved change.

But when I compare a nurse's salary with those of other professionals, accountants for example, an unfair discrepancy still exists. I went to school as long as an accountant; I passed exams just as demanding and difficult. If he makes a mistake it could cost you a couple of thousand dollars or, if he makes a serious mistake, it could cost your entire business. If I made a mistake as a nurse, it could prolong your hospital stay and possibly cause some physical damage, but if I make a serious mistake, I could kill you.

But in our value system nurses make very low income in proportion to accountants.

However, the increase in nurses' pay has developed situations in which I have heard nurses say "If it's a choice between buying better treatment equipment, or something else, I'd rather see my pay check be increased." Or, "I work at this hospital instead of the other, simply because I make more money here."

I thank God this attitude is applicable only to a fairly small proportion of nurses. Most are still working dedicated service oriented lives.

A lot of us prefer to work at a certain hospital because its goals match our goals and our interests in quality care are the same. So I consider myself more of the old school than the modern school, although I am still in my thirties. We were taught that you don't waste supplies. You don't use an extra syringe unless absolutely necessary. You watch the hospital's budget instead of your own and try to avoid extra costs for the patient.

I also feel very strongly that the patient should be trained to care for himself as much as possible . . . and the family be encouraged to help too.

I've worked in many departments in many hospitals, geographically scattered, due to my husband's frequent moves. I've worked in critical care, in pediatrics, in the emergency room and have seen a reoccurring situation . . . pushing a family aside and even limiting their visiting hours. What should we permit?

It annoys me and many family members of patients that, after an individual has been cared for lovingly by a family member, perhaps for nearly a lifetime, one of my sister nurses wants to take over and treat that patient almost by herself, very possessively. We can understand that dedication, but the family must be permitted to be around. Not to permit their visits at almost any time is simply not fair—and maybe not best for the patient.

I once worked in a hospital where there was a lot of dissension and negativism. The nurses came from all over the country, from good hospitals, each having different treatment techniques and many different state laws. Each nurse had been trained and knew what to do—back home—and any other procedure was just wrong.

We had to face the fact that many or most of those nurses were facing different legal requirements, something of which the public is usually unaware. The nursing administration in this hospital wasn't sufficiently strong to control the situation which had been doing on for a number of years and was eroding patient care.

Sometimes this situation led to comments by the public like "Don't go over there for treatment; they don't know what they are doing."

When I left that hospital, the situation was completely reversed. We had begun to realize that we were a team, agreement on procedures being the only way we could accomplish the goals we faced.

From this came my philosophy for a hospital, or any organization, which is:

> If the hospital's goals are not
> my goals, or if I cannot be
> supportive of those goals, then
> I'm not necessarily a bad
> person—but I don't belong as
> a member of this hospital

Yes, this resulted in some turnover which, in the long run, was beneficial to all concerned.

We were a for-profit organization, privately owned, and did not accept government funding. Therefore we didn't have to provide a lot of care to indigent people. Many people, who had never worked in this type of institution, found circumstances completely foreign to them.

This hospital gradually regained its prestigious position in the community and was able to meet its two major goals, i.e. first, to provide the best possible patient care and, second, to meet the profit goal of its stockholders.

Today, small hospitals such as that one, because of the nature of Medicare/Medicaid are closing all over the country. They do not have enough commercial business to keep their doors open. In this area the high average age and the huge numbers of Medicare patients create an abnormal situation, dangerous economically to the hospital.

We nurses have to be idealistic but we must deal with the realistic also. If we only live in clouds, we cannot deal with what's here in the real world.

RN
Name withheld on request
Florida

NURSING CAN BE EXCITING

Many people don't think of nursing as an exciting career but, believe me, it is. My experiences as a crical care nurse have proven them wrong. Some of the most exciting, challenging situations are those that involve human life, illness and death and people's responses to them. One's emotions as the caregiver of a critically ill person run the gamut from laughter at the inside jokes told by the staff to excitement during an emergency, to depression from the quick letdown when a crisis suddenly ends. I experienced all of these when a patient, Mrs. Hansen, had open heart surgery.

She arrived in SICU (surgical intensive care unit) cold, pale, bloated, and entangled in invasive monitoring lines. Large diameter drainage tubes emerged from the chest. Several intravenous lines were in the arms infusing blood and fluids. Open heart patients cannot speak because of a breathing tube placed in the trachea, but can probably hear much of what is going on around them. The nurses hooked up the lines and monitors, restored order to the incomprehensible tangle of tubes, and quickly assessed the patient. Was she getting enough oxygen? Was she bleeding excessively? Had she developed any blood clots? Was her heart pumping effectively? Did she need more fluid? Was she waking up yet? Was her family nearby?

As this process occurred, the SICU resident lingered at the foot of the bed waiting for "the numbers," which is the list of heart pressures gleaned from various monitoring lines and verified by the nurse. The resident looked them over, confident that he would be alerted if there were any other problems. Confidence in Gini, the nurse caring for this patient, was paramount to this resident who had not yet done his cardiothoracic rotating. The patient had a quiet night.

Gini cared for Mrs. Hansen again the next day. Her progress was not stellar, but nothing pointed to a crisis. Gini began to notice climbing heart pressures as she bathed her patient. When she called the resident, Bill Butrich, she had already turned off the nitroprusside and nitroglycerine intravenous drips, two potent vasodilators.

Mrs. Hansen's blood pressure was 89/64. Combined with chest tube outputs and high heart pressures, a low blood pressure is an ominous sign. Mrs. Hansen's blood pressure dropped to zero, but there was still a pattern on the cardiac monitor. Gini called for help and started CPR (cardiopulmonary resuscitation) I responded from the next room. Knowing Bill would not open the chest himself, as is necessary to do proper CPR on an open heart patient, I shouted to the secretary to call the chief resident. I gloved, gowned, and masked, and prepared the sterile open chest tray of instruments. Standing there waiting for the resident seemed like hours. The thought passed through my head, as it had before, that I could do it. Just crack the chest myself, zip the incision open with a scalpel, snip the wires securing the breastbone, insert the rib spreaders, and I'd be in. Other nurses buzzed around the room, preparing medications, taking turns at writing down each step of the resuscitation process. The resident arrived, opened the chest, and found a bleeding vessel filling the sack around the heart with blood, compressing the heart. He put a finger over the vessel and we ran to the operating room. The resident had both hands inside the open chest, running clumsily alongside the bed with the respiratory therapist, Gini, and me. Someone cracked a joke about the resident's "Polish CPR" and light laughter followed to relieve the tense situation briefly.

Outside the operating room, Gini and I collected the SICU equipment and walked back downstairs. Still high from the adrenalin rush of an open chest, we chattered about what led to the arrest, how smoothly the open chest effort went, how the patient looked, whether we thought she'd live. But, by the time we walked down the single flight of stairs, there was little conversation left. Gini would have to get ready for the return of a very critical patient in case the patient lived, and I had another patient to care for. Time was too short to rehash the experience. Yet I felt a need to tell someone about what we had just done: a magnificent team effort put forth, about transporting the patient to the OR (operating room) in record time, about how we might have saved her life. But Gini already knew all this, so we re-entered the SICU in silence, drained.

(Ed.: I cannot help noticing how similar was their reaction to success as would be a sports team which came from behind to win, or a marketing team that achieved great success in introducing a new product. These two nurses had reason to be proud.)

Many of my memories are snapshots of patients whose names I remember, and maybe a few other details, but the most distinct memories are of the emotions those people engendered in me.

I felt hopelessness looking at Mrs. K. with 13 intravenous pumps regularly infusing 13 different drugs and fluids into her, a wide open infected abdominal wound, an arteriovenous shunt in her bloated arm connected to a cylindrical filter substituting for her failed kidneys, a ventilator hooked to her tracheostomy because she was too weak to breathe on her own.

She was too weak and demented from a long ICU stay to communicate in writing. Yet her anxious family was frightened of putting an end to these extraordinary efforts because they had invested so much love and concern that they needed to believe she would recover. They didn't have the benefit of the nurse's multiple experiences with patients on a slow downhill course that will inevitably end in death. This allowed them to cling to the shreds of hope brought about by her opening her eyes part way, or trying to move her restrained arm. They looked to me for reassurance that they should find hope in these acts, and I experienced a familiar dilemma. Should I encourage the hope that they desperately needed to cope with this tragedy, while keeping them rooted in the reality of the patient's condition?

Some nurses must leave the room when the family visits because they know their cynicism would come through in such encounters. It is a hard thing to do—to balance what you know to be true, but can't say, with what you think you should say, but which isn't true. I cope by choosing my words very carefully, by using my verbal skills to walk the thin line that allows me to help the family in the way they want to be helped and the way I know I should.

Mrs. K. finally died after three surgeries, a long line of invasive procedures, literally hundreds of IV bags and tubings, and seven primary nurses. It is hard for a seasoned nurse to accept the magnificant high-technology efforts put forth for an elderly cancer stricken woman with a weak heart, then admit a fifty-year old man who's having a stroke because he stopped taking the blood pressure medication he couldn't afford. It is exhilarating to know that I can help

both of these patients and their families, but hard to accept the paradoxes brought about by a system that encourages cure over care.
Teresa Tarnowski Goodell, RN, BSN, CCRN
Lorain, Ohio

MY PATIENT WAS TARGETED FOR A HIT

I had just received notice that I had passed state boards after waiting agonizing weeks.

I was scheduled for second shift that day as a staff nurse in the medical-surgical intensive care unit of a large metropolitan county hospital.

As I arrived at work I was elated. Finally I was an RN. Those years of preparation had paid off and I could now sign in as an RN instead of an SN or GN.

The patient to whom I was assigned was a gentleman who had been shot earlier that day but who was now stabilized. I was confident I could take care of him competently but, as I received report from the off-going nurse I learned there was more to the story than I had been told.

It seems the man who had shot my patient was now in jail but his relatives were coming from a nearby city to finish the job.

I froze. Nothing like this had been covered in school. I had psychosocial skills but this seemed overwhelming. Was I to have studied all these years only to be shot in the cross-fire? Me—an RN for only six hours?

But my peers were supportive. Local police were informed of the situation and my patient's name was removed from any place where the public might have access to it. The doors of the unit were kept closed. Any time those doors were opened I jumped two feet.

The night wore on. My patient was stable and I thought maybe I would be an RN longer than one day. Two more hours into the shift I received a telephone call. Two detectives were in the emergency room and would like to come up to ask my patient a few questions.

Now my observation and assessment skills would have to be at top level. I had to be certain these men were really detectives and not cleverly disguised.

The door opened and two men dressed in suits walked in. They were stopped by another nurse for whom they produced proper identification. They had passed checkpoint!

As they walked into my patient's room I was hanging an intravenous bag. I turned and prayed silently that my dreams of becoming a caring, knowledgeable nurse would not be short-lived. The two men showed me their badges and explained their intentions.

After making sure their actions would not be endangering to my patient I left the room. I probably could have floated out that door—I was so happy I was given the opportunity to practice as an RN for one more shift anyway.

Patricia Volkert, RN
West Allis, Wisconsin

PEOPLE DIDN'T TREAT PETER NORMALLY

I was a young nurse who had worked only two years full time with the public health nursing department in a midwestern town. We provided emotional and physical support for families with special needs. I was 23 years old and, to say the least, was very inexperienced in nursing and in life.

A referral came from the state university concerning a five year old boy named Peter who had been diagnosed as having a degenerative brain disorder of unknown etiology. He had developed normally until at age five he started regressing slowly, step by step. In this process of regressing he seizured almost continuously. However, this spirited little boy still attempted to smile between seizures.

On my second visit to Peter's family, the mother was cleaning her cupboards and Peter was on a blanket in the kitchen watching her. I remember thinking "Why would she be cleaning cupboards when this child is in such need of her constant attention?" I picked up the boy, and rocked him and started singing while the mother continued to work.

In the midst of my singing she stopped cleaning and started crying. She sat beside me and wept for nearly ten minutes. At first I thought I had done something to offend her but that was not the case at all.

She offered me some Russian tea and told me her sad story.

Since Peter had started seizuring, people were afraid to hold him or even talk to him. It was as if he weren't Peter anymore. I was the first person to pick him up spontaneously and treat him normally. The mother said she needed to see that more than anything else . . . being so hurt by society's turning its back on the boy.

We talked for over an hour about the problems of having a chronically ill child, and how it affected the whole family. Her faith had been tested over and over again.

Three years later my own first child was born with cerebral palsy and was retarded. He also had seizures. After my initial shock I thought of Peter. I telephoned his mother to tell her I now knew exactly how she had felt and I thanked her for teaching me to share and express my feelings with others. I knew from my experience with Peter that uncomfortable feelings need to be dealt with or they become hidden problems. The best advice Peter's mother gave me was to write a diary of my feelings and emotions. I kept one for five years; now, each time I look at it I think how, through an odd twist of fate, my life has somewhat paralleled their story.

Now my son is 16 and has moved into a group home with other retarded teenagers. We have sold our home which we built for him 12 years ago so he could stay where he was raised. The diary I kept for those beginning years was a godsend and I will be eternally grateful to this lady who was Peter's mother.

Jo Augustine, RN
Rochester, MN

MY BRAIN-DEAD PATIENT

One night I was working in intensive care caring for an 18 year old young man who had suffered a severe head injury in a motor vehicle crash. His brain injury was catastrophic and he had been given maximal treatment, without result. Part of this treatment included barbiturate coma. In this therapy, patients are given very high doses of barbiturates in an effort to slow the metabolism of the brain and to make the brain more resistant to damage. Unfortunately, this therapy so suppresses the brain that the patient appears dead.

The patient did poorly and was believed to be brain dead by the physician and nurses. The barbiturate therapy was stopped and we prepared to pronounce the patient brain dead. However, a patient cannot be declared brain dead if he has high levels of barbiturates in his blood because this can cause the patient to appear brain dead even though he is not. Measurement of the patient's blood levels showed that he did indeed have too much barbiturate in his blood to allow pronouncement of death. Thus we had a patient whom all of us believed to be brain dead, whose heart and lungs were functioning well, and whom we had to leave on the ventilator because his lab values would not allow him to be disconnected.

Shortly after my shift began that night I met this young man's parents. They were obviusly well educated and fully understood the paradox of the situation. Frequently during the early part of my shift they would visit. Father would stand at the bedside, stroking his son and looking at his unmarked yet dead face. In the early morning father came to visit his son while mom slept. As my work was caught up, I too stood at the bedside while father and I talked. He told me that his son had been a model child, that he had never been trouble to his parents. The father was obviously proud of his son. Equally obvious was that the father fully realized that his son was dead; he even spoke of him in the past tense. The father was quite clearly a kind, caring, loving man who was tormented by the legal conundrum trapping his son.

As we talked he told me of a incident that had happened in this same hospital, in which a nurse was believed to have intentionally hastened a patient's death with a common electrolyte solution. I had previously heard bits and pieces of this story and knew it to be a tender, sensitive situation. He told me that even after the nurse had confessed, the district attorney's office chose not to prosecute, because there was no physical evidence. He said the physical evidence was lacking because potassium chloride is normally found in great quantity inside cells and after death that potassium is released into the body fluids. Thus, at autopsy, the coroner would only find the normally elevated levels of potassium in the body. Thus, without evidence, the case would have been lost in court.

After the father told me this story he told me how difficult the current situation was for his wife. She loved her son very much and the ambiguity and the wait for the inevitable was tormenting her almost more than she could take. It seemed so pointless, albeit logical, to have to spend days waiting for the son's laboratory values to change, when he was obviously dead. At this point they had been waiting several days for the barbiturate level to drop off.

After this wrenching discussion, emphasizing the fact that my patient was already dead except for signing the papers, plus the difficulties the authorities had prosecuting a nurse in this very unit for her actions, and the torment that the waiting was for mother and father, the father made one parting comment. He looked straight into my eyes and said "You know, Jim, it would be so much easier for us if he just died tonight." I did not challenge this statement, nor did I ask for clarification.

His meaning was clear. What I was to do was not clear.

This incident occurred a long time ago in another state. I think it reads better if I do not tell what decision I made, nor what I did. I will simply say that I sleep quite well every night.

I only want the reader to understand that this event did not happen in the facility where I now work. Not even in this city.

James P. McGraw, RN, MN, CCRN, CEN
Fort Worth, Texas

THOSE HUGS AND THANKS

In 39 years of active nursing there have been numerous highs and lows. However, it is many little things that stay in one's memory bank . . . going all the way back to student days.

When you are afraid of the good doctors and one day you are sought out by one of the most eminent surgeons and expect to be reprimanded — only to be told that you were the only one who had applied a hot compress the exact way he had ordered it. It was an encouraging word of praise and greatly appreciated.

It is the moments of sitting with a family of a terminal patient and being told it felt good having you there.

My last years of work were spent in an OB/GYN clinic where there was litle hands-on dealing with critically ill patients, but long listening/talking sessions with patients and families who have lost a baby through a miscarriage or because of some other tragedy.

And there was the hug that came after you could tell someone who had gone through months of infertility studies that her pregnancy test was finally positive.

It is those hugs and those "Thank yous" that made my job the great pleasure it has been.

RN
Name withheld by request
Oshkosh, Wisconsin

SALLY'S LAST WEEK

The phone rang.

"Sally is vomiting and doesn't want to return to the hospital. The doctor said that if someone can put in an IV, she can stay home."

I knew my new neighbor had cancer and didn't have long to live. But I didn't know anything about what it meant to Sally and her family until I received that telephone call.

Sally's cancer began with a lump in her breast six years previously when she and her husband were missionaries in South America. Over the next few years Sally had several surgery procedures and many series of radiation and chemotherapy treatment. A remission at one point had given hope for a miracle but it didn't last. Now there was metastasis to the brain and spinal cord.

When she first became ill, her mother-in-law, known as Granny Liz, came to live with the family. Sally remained in charge of the family but Granny Liz assisted with the cleaning, laundry, meals and child care. The three children, Judy, 14, Philip, 13, and Carrie, 11, had grown up having a sick mother.

I agreed to insert the IV so Sally wouldn't have to leave her family and go to the hospital which was seventy miles away. Her doctor called the local hospital pharmacy and I picked up the solution and tubing on my way home from work that evening. I asked a nurse friend, Muriel, who lived nearby, to assist me.

We inserted the IV, improvising a drapery rod for an IV pole.

During the night Sally's friend watched the IV but called me in the early morning when the IV had infiltrated. I rushed over to discontinue it. The Compazine and Dilaudid we had given Sally had taken effect and she was sleeping, so I decided against reinserting the IV. Later in the morning I talked with her doctor who said the IV was no longer needed since Sally was not vomiting and had started taking fluids orally.

A few days later Sally went to the hospital for the usual tests. The impression was that she would not be coming home. When I visited her that weekend she was considerably weaker. As I helped her to the bathroom she said "I didn't know anyone could be so weak." I was sure I had seen her for the last time.

I was wrong! She had a strong desire to be with her family when she died. With no available home health care in her community, her wish didn't seem possible. However, the family got a commitment from Muriel and me to assist with the nursing care. An LPN, a close family friend who lived nearby, said she would also help. She gave the general nursing care—bathing, skin care, enemas, etc. Every day Sally insisted she get into the bathtub and then dress in a beautiful nightgown. Sh liked pretty things and insisted that she be well-groomed and well-dressed.

Muriel and I gave all the injections and managed the care. We talked with her doctor to receive orders and to make sure we had not overlooked any aspect of her care. We also spoke with the nurse who had supervised her care in the hospital. We made arrangements to get blood work done.

We set up a notebook as an informal chart to record vital signs, observations and medications. This became confusing at times because Sally was accustomed to taking medications on her own. She would take medication and forget to tell us; we were always in danger of giving her too much analgesic or antiemetic. This was especially true when she began to be semi-comatose. We finally had to remove the medications from her bedside. I hated to see her lose that independence but it just wasn't safe anymore.

She lived only one more week.

During her last week friends and relatives came from all over the country to say goodbye. The house was constantly filled with people, conversation and love. Although the children had seemed ill at ease at the hospital with their mother, at home they resumed their normal activities of school and play and spent time with their mother when she was awake.

And Sally continued to direct the household affairs.

"Sally, where are those jeans we bought for the girls? I can hem them for you now."

"Did we write a check for that last MasterCharge bill?"

Part of our involvement included the family's growing acceptance of Sally's death. Having her at home during this last week helped Sally's husband, Bob, accept that she would not get well. He was devastated. Every night until the very last weekend Sally and Bob slept arm-in-arm. At first I felt like an intruder when I went in each morning to give Sally's cortisone injection. I knew their marriage had been a rewarding one. They had always worked together, first as missionaries and now in a local church. Bob was losing his partner, confidante and closest friend.

We tried to help Sally conserve her energy so she could accomplish all her goals that week. She spent her waking hours with friends and making tapes for her children. She told each the history of their life from the moment each was placed on her stomach by the physician. Bob's tape was personal and loving, chronicling their life together.

NURSE

She became comatose that last weekend, so we rented a hospital bed and inserted a Foley catheter. A nurse friend came for the weekend and wanted to care for her. Muriel and I were on call.

Monday morning I came over to give the usual injections; as I started to turn her comatose body over I realized she wasn't breathing. I listened with my stethoscope to confirm what I knew was true; Sally was dead. She must have just died a few minutes before I arrived.

My work as a volunteer nurse was over. Sally had left directions for all the arrangements for her funeral. As the family began planning I found myself wanting to help but nursing care was why I was there and it was no longer needed. This family was in its own home. There was no hospital paper work to deal with, no morgue care to give, no husband grieving alone with the rest of the family miles away. The whole family was there and could support each other. I was in the way.

Then I found a task I could do. The dress Sally had wanted to wear at the funeral was dirty, so I carried the dress to the cleaners, the last task I could do to close this experience for me.

Providing home care to Sally was a rewarding, yet exhausting learning experience for me. While everything didn't go as smoothly as I wanted, there is no doubt in my mind that home care was best for Sally and her family. The patient had known what was best for her!

Providing home care for those patients who choose to die at home is one of the greatest challenges we face.

Judy R. Thorson, RN
Omaha, Nebraska

THE COUNTRY WOMAN

I work in a 1600 bed hospital in a large city. Many of our patients are referred to our facility from the surrounding rural areas. Granny Perkins, a 74-year-old patient with heart disease was referred for evaluation of her irregular heart rhythm from a small town in the country, by her local internal medicine physician. The tests recommended were very complicated—an electrophysiologic study and a cardiac catheterization.

The first day of hospitalization I introduced myself as a nurse researcher and welcomed her to our hospital. I explained to her that I would be seeing her daily as a patient educator. I added that my job was to explain all scheduled procedures to her and to answer any questions she may have. Every day I visited Granny and attempted to explain in lay terms what to expect during her hospitalization. She generally was very noncommittal and stared out the window. During most visits she would point to the pigeons outside roosting on the ledge of the hospital and comment that if she had her gun with her, she would shoot a few to make a pie. I worried that she was frightened and not comprehending her situation. I couldn't help but feel I was not reaching her. At times I even felt she really did not know who I was, in spite of the fact that she was hospitalized for several weeks and saw me frequently. I rationalized that a country woman and a city woman probably had little in common. Soon after she was discharged from the hospital, I received the following letter that made me realize she certainly did know who I was and had a great sense of humor as well.

"Dear Dr. Porterfield: I'm doing just fine. I'm sending some more money from Medicare. Next Saturday is my birthday. I'll be sixteen years old. Ha! Ha! I'm looking for a present from you. Granny Perkins."

Now I find comfort in the fact that although my patients don't always acknowledge my presence, I still may be making a positive impact on their lives and maybe even a new friend. I sent her a birthday card and note.

Linda Porterfield, RN, PhD
Memphis, Tennessee

A GOOD SENSE OF HUMOR

One day I was caring for a C.O.P.D. (chronic obstructive pulmonary disease) patient who had a great sense of humor.

I ran a rhythm strip early in the morning when I came on shift and noticed later, about 10:30 A.M., that his electrocardiogram (ECG) had changed in appearance.

Since I was planning to bathe him I went in to check on his lead wires and chest electrodes. While checking the wires I noticed that the negative (white) lead was not in its correct position. I followed the wire down from the monitoring juncture and found the patch with the lead wire intact stuck to the patient's scrotum.

You can imagine the patient's and my surprise when we found the patch's resting place.

As I mentioned, this patient had an extremely good sense of humor. While I dissolved in fits of laughter, he said "I guess they were trying to monitor any activity down there."

By that time we were both laughing and I was sprawled at the edge of the bed too weak to get up.

Laurie A. Johnson, RN
Omaha, Nebraska

SPECIAL PATIENTS

Four years ago we admitted an eighteen-year-old boy who had been seriously injured in an ATV (all terrain vehicle) accident. His pelvis was fragmented, his buttocks were literally exploded, and he had severe internal injuries. He required a colostomy and developed ARDS (acute respiratory distress syndrome) requiring long-term ventilator management.

The radial nerve in his left arm was destroyed, causing that extremity to be paralyzed. Due to the severe injuries to his buttocks and pelvis he developed gas gangrene in one leg and needed surgery, which damaged the sciatic nerve, causing near-paralysis in that leg.

His biggest problem, however, was the raw, open tissue of his buttocks. Despite everything, he frequently began hemorrhaging from that area and needed blood transfusions, pressure packs, etc. to control the bleeding and to keep him alive.

Even though he was young, coherent and fighting to survive, the physicians said there was no way he could make it, due to the hemorrhaging which occurred one to three times each twenty-four hour period. The nurses kept transfusing him and trying every possible way to stop the bleeding. Finally a surgeon made one more attempt to cauterize the wound and it worked.

The patient eventually came off the ventilator, began eating and started rehabilitation. He not only survived but is able to walk now. If the nurses had given up when some of the doctors did, however, he never would have made it. I was very proud to be a part of such a dedicated group.

Just two years ago we admitted a patient to ICU (intensive care unit) who had come in by taxi and told the emergency room nurse that he was going into CHF (congestive heart failure). Although he was initially stable, he had an extensive cardiac history, and was in the process of trying to raise enough money for a heart transplant.

I took care of him and, sure enough, he went into full-blown pulmonary edema. We controlled it but he also had problems with cardiac arrhythmias due to his cardiomyopathy. He was on medication for these, but still frequently had runs of ventricular tachycardia, which would convert (stop itself) spontaneously.

He was transferred to telemetry where I kept track of him. Forty-eight hours after his transfer I was working in ICU when a cardiac arrest code (alarm) was called in his room. An ICU nurse usually responds to codes in other areas and I think I broke a speed record getting to his room. There I found CPR (cardiopulmonary resuscitation) in progress, but no doctor, no supervisor yet. I ran the code, defibrillating and ordering drugs. (Ed.: By "running the code" the nurse means she was following the procedures as dictated in her standing orders.) By the time the ER staff could get there the patient was out of danger and required only one more shock to convert his heart. Back we went to ICU. He did not wake up for twenty-four hours, until I came back on duty. At this point he was accepted for an emergency heart transplant and left us.

I was scared to death, but remembered what to do and ran a textbook code, saving this man's life. (Ed.: She is saying she followed standing orders and that everything went perfectly). He did receive his transpant and I believe still resides somewhere in Michigan.

Our standard introduction to a patient when we come on duty is "My name is Mary and I'll be taking care of you until eleven tonight." Usually that is all there is to it, but not always. One night a patient replied "I'm hurt" so I asked "What's wrong?" He said "Nothing, my name is Hurt."

Another patient beat me to the punch by saying immediately I entered. "Hi. My name is Bill Smith and I'll be your patient to night." It gave the entire night a lighter note.

Mary S. Gulbrandsen, RN, BSN, CCRN
Lake Worth, Florida

OUTREACH NURSE SCORES AGAIN

I am an Outreach Nurse, doing case management and home care for an over-65 population. Nurses usually are pleased with any positive outcome but there is something specially valuable about the recognition inherent in an unsolicited testimonial from the patient himself.

Recently a patient of mine wrote to my department manager, sending the following letter, which is very dear and very much appreciated by me. It was sent to the Senior Plan Office manager of our unit.

"I don't know whether I can find the right words to tell you how much I appreciate the fine things that my senior plan outreach nurse has done for me and is still continuing to do. Her name is CJ Burrell and she has been coming to see me every Tuesday morning at 8:30 A.M. She tests my blood sugar, my blood pressure, my pulse and temperature. She then examines my feet and fills my syringes for the coming week. You see, I am a diabetic and my vision is very poor. I also need a cane to walk without falling. The fact that I know that I will have someone coming to test my sugar keeps me from eating those things that I should avoid. I try to be careful and the result is that my diabetes had been under good control. My doctor just told me that I am his number one diabetic patient, for which I thank my nurse.

"I have something else to thank her for. Last May I became ill on a Saturday and I felt awful. Sunday was no better and I stayed in bed all that day too. On Monday I felt just a little better but far from all right and when CJ showed up on Tuesday she was aghast. She thought I looked terrible and then she saw my leg. It was discolored and mottled and was very badly infected. She called my doctor who sent an ambulance to rush me to the hospital. He was waiting for me and I was admitted and an IV program was started. I was there for six days and was completely cured.

"Later my doctor told me that had treatment been delayed for another 48 hours I would probably have lost my leg. I will never be able to thank CJ for her expertise in recognizing what was wrong and in taking quick action. I owe her my leg and probably my life. I have, from time to time, had other outreach nurses who have helped. There was Fran Fowler, of whom I am very fond, Janet Block, Bonnie, and some whose names escape me at the moment.

"What I am trying to bring out is that this program is so fantastic not only for me but for the countless others who need and benefit from it. These ladies are like a ray of sunshine in the bleak of night. They make a big difference in the quality of health many of us seniors rely on . All I can say is keep up the wonderful work you do. The hospital must be very proud of all of you."

(Ed.: I have seen the original of this letter but choose not to reveal the name of the writer.)

CJ Burrell, RN, C.
Honolulu, Hawaii

I THANK GOD FOR YOU EVERY NIGHT

In May, 1988, I was a nurse working in the extremely busy coronary care unit at a large hospital in Philadelphia, Pennsylvania.

One of my primary patients, Antonio Prestini, had suffered several myocardial infarctions, resulting in severe cardiac damage. After one of his many cardiac arrests, he ended up orally intubated and on a ventilator. (Ed.: a tube had been introduced into his trachea and oxygen was being supplied.)

Throughout the three weeks he was a patient in our unit, his wife of 47 years faithfully visited him every single day, a difficult trip in a large city.

On May 21, at 7 o'clock at night, Mr. Prestini extubated himself (removed his own breathing tube) and the medical staff elected not to replace it. He stabilized quickly and began to talk about his frustrations and fears of the intensive care setting. Around 9 o'clock I decided to take the portable telephone to his bedside so he could communicate with his devoted wife. He anxiously dialed the number and talked with his wife for several minutes.

At 10:30 that same night he decompensated rapidly (Ed.: the heart lost its ability to maintain adequate circulation) and he went into cardiac arrest again. After a long time of very intensive therapy, the code was terminated and he was pronounced dead.

Two months later, after the emotional period has passed, I received a letter from Mrs. Prestini. Here are some excerpts from that letter, detailing her feelings:

"For months I have thought of you, the nurse whose kindness was unforgettable. You did something I will never forget and I will always be grateful. You connected an extension phone so I could speak with my husband. It was the last time because he died suddenly in late evening that May 21.

"It was most difficult accepting his sudden death, but I received some solace from having had the chance to wish him a good night's sleep and to tell him I loved him. For 47 years we had never retired without saying that to each other.

"Saying thank you cannot express the depth of my appreciation.

However, since that night, not a day goes by that I have not thanked God for your goodness and kindness. God bless you."

I guess you never realize the importance of even the simplest tasks we do that can make such an impression on someone. This experience truly expresses the reason I chose a career in nursing.

Catherine P. Lovecchio, RN
Lewisburg, Pennsylvania

CAN DEATH BE BEAUTIFUL?

This event made me realize that a moment of sorrow can also be a moment of joy.

I have been a nurse for 14 years, always working the acute care setting. Many times I have been present during the expiration of a patient, sometimes unexpected, sometimes not. Sometimes traumatic to the patient, as in a code situation, sometimes quietly in the wee hours of the night with family unaware or not present.

Recently I experienced a patient's demise which was filled with peace, joy and love.

The patient, a male, had been critically ill for several weeks and chronically ill for a year. During the night his respiratory status deteriorated and by early morning it was evident he would not survive the day without immediate intervention of life-support procedures.

His family was called and were there within minutes—two daughters and his wife.

As he became unresponsive and his heart rate dropped they quickly decided to let him go peacefully. Holding his hands and stroking his face, they gently, verbally led him toward death, thanking him for his love as a father and a husband and reassuring him. They told him it was all right to go and that they would all meet again "in the garden."

Within a minute he had expired surrounded with the love of his family.

After numerous dealings with the death of patients, this one will forever be etched in my mind as being beautiful, if death can be referred to as such.

I was proud and enlightened to be an RN here in the face of tragedy.

Staria R. Ferreira, RN
Palm Desert, CA

A FIGHT FOR LIFE

I have many stories but I choose to tell you about a little child that was born at Children's Hospital. Joshua was a term baby who, after he was born, all we could find that was wrong physiologically, was a very large tongue. But this very large tongue would keep falling back and blocking the esophagus. So the only way that Joshua could breathe was sitting up — a totally upright position. I mean almost a traction on a tongue, the poor little guy. As long as we could keep his tongue forward, he was fine.

Finally, after about a week of this, we figured that we would have to let the traction off and find what next to do. So we did. To our shock and surprise he never had any more problems. He had what we call apnea and bradycardia. He would stop breathing and his heart would stop or slow down. He had no more of these spells. Then we moved into other problems with him. He started having feeding problems, meaning that we would feed him and sometimes, unexpectedly, he would immediately throw up everything he had eaten. Needless to say, the only time he would eat well was when I would feed him. We did what we called primary nursing at that time and I became Joshua's primary nurse. When you are in primary nursing or similar specialty units, you become very close to the family also. I did with his family. He was their second child.

Well, Joshua is now a couple of months old; he still is in the hospital and is growing, but feeding problems are still an issue. Then he started to have what we thought was a seizure. We weren't really sure. We didn't have MRI (Ed.; magnetic resonance imaging) at that time but we did a cat scan, and they found a questionable growth on his brain stem. Once they saw that, they figured it probably explained the throwing up and the questionable seizures. So, what they did, after a lot of emotional discussions with all the staff and the family, was what was similar to an angiogram, a test where they were going to inject some dye. There were some risks, even the possibility that Joshua might die, because we didn't really know what was the problem. The parents were well aware of this and took the chance.

They did the tests. I was working nights that week and I knew that when I came in that night, I'd know how things went. I had been visiting friends that night, not too far from the hospital. I no sooner got into the unit than people started saying "Kathy, we've been trying to locate you. Joshua is not doing well." Not laying guilt on me, they just wanted me to know that things weren't going well. Remember that I was still his primary nurse after two months or so, a big assignment. I stopped to visit Josh for just a few moments and said I'd be back at eleven. I visited my friends and they said they'd help me get ready for the return to Joshua. That wasn't the plan of the evening, but that is what happened.

I was really glad that I knew that he was not doing well because it gave me time to acquire strength before I returned, because I am a person who, in a crisis, performs well, but I fall apart afterwards. I work with some people who fall apart in a crisis and are totally dysfunctional, but I do my falling apart afterwards. I get through the crisis and then I deal with the aftermath.

We dealt with Joshua but we knew that he was dying. Of course at that age, two months, a child doesn't know what is happening.

His family had chosen to go home to sleep because I was there. They said they felt that the person who could deal best with Joshua in his dying hours was me and, besides, they had a slightly older girl at home who needed love and family presence. So they chose to go home. Of course they had already had two months of living hell and it was now eleven at night. There was nothing they could do anyhow. It was around 2 A.M. and I had been talking to Josh all this time, telling him things that were going on, telling him that I loved him, as did many others. Then he opened his eyes. It was obvious that he knew exactly who I was. We had about two very brief moments, actually two minutes, when his eyes were open and he heard every word I had just said. Then he closed them and he proceeded to die.

Everyone—the nurses and the doctors—were very supportive of

me. They knew how attached I had become to Josh and that it was like losing my own chid.

His mom and dad had called in a couple of times and knew that the end was near. They helped us make the decision to let him go, no more drugs. So we kept the respirator on and I just sat and rocked him. The family was called and realized they could not make it before he took his last breath. They knew that I was holding him, rocking him, and that is what he needed.

They had had their time with him, but it is hard, very hard. The parents and I are still friends and see each other frequently.

When they came in we had disconnected all the tubes and things and they had only to deal with Joshua. So they spent time with him, perhaps as long as two hours. I really believe we should let people have time with the dead. Probably the one that struck me the most was the grandpa who talked about the dreams he had for his grandson, how he wanted to go fishing, to teach the boy how to play ball. It actually helped the mother and dad in their grief problems.

I was doing quite well until I touched a blanket I had made for him. Then I literally fell apart.

What's interesting about this reaction is this is not what you expect from a nurse, or from a doctor.

To this day we still communicate. Both of the parents found that they have a genetic malfunction in producing males. If they produce girls they are okay, but in producing males they have a problem. They now have two girls, one older and one younger than Josh.

Another piece of this story is that five years later I had moved out of that section and had moved into obstetrical care at another large hospital. Josh's mother's sister came in, in labor and was told by Josh's mother "Trust her. She'll help you through any problems." She also birthed a premature infant without any problems, but she had total trust in me. Still she had the potential of inherited problem genes but, thank God, everything went fine. She wouldn't do anything without discussing it with me. Of course it is nice to have that referred love. All she wanted was to have me tell her all the risks and not to worry too much about the possible congenital problems. Females appear to have a number of genetic malfunctions that never surface so if there is any sort of malfunction in the family, in recent years we go increasingly to genetic testing. So she had a very healthy little girl.

Life does have interlocking situations.

Kathy Kerber, RN, MS
Clinical Nurse Specialist
Minneapolis, MN

MY MOTHER IS COMING TOMORROW

I've filled a legal pad with scribblings and scratchings yet I find it hard to order my impressions. I now sit here, a teacher of 15 years, my head spinning after a day in my new career as a hospital nurse. Images whirl through my mind—both too awful and too awesome to bring into focus. Fragments of the day's work form and reform in momentary patterns behind my closed eyelids, becoming a kaleidoscope of contradictions.

I see blood red, urine yellow, bruise blue, necrotic black—bits of this and that align. Smashed skulls, stapled backs, shaved heads, curved incisions, bandage turbans, surgical drains, crani caps and new toupees. Wincing and whining, whistling in the dark, tears, dogged determination, confusion and withdrawal, anxiety so strong it quakes the whole being and sends after-shocks as well, trusting surrender—all witnessed in a typical day.

The unfairness of disease and accident is a striking contrast. I have stood in the hall and felt the very air sucked out of the room as the neurosurgeons exit. The weight of mortality descends upon a new mother, a beloved grandparent or a recently exuberant teen, and I mourn for the lost illusions. Why, I wonder, did I ever want a job that was "real" and honest? Yet, I know when I move a few feet away I hear the promises of tumors removed, pain numbed, eyesight saved, walking restored. The dive into sorrow and soaring with elation make for a dizzying change, but I prefer it to numbness.

This hospital draws staff and patients from all over the world. The spirit of the heroic doctors and the compassionate sisters is a discernible presence. Patients come with hope—a hog farmer from Iowa, a teacher from South Dakota, a butcher from Argentina, a

71

CEO from Chicago, a retired mortician from Minnesota, a prince from Saudi Arabia, a judge from Kansas, an heiress from Italy, with poets, truckers, doctors, prisoners and presidents. We ease them out of the mink coats, the overalls, the three-piece suits, the Amish sus-pendered pants, the desert robes, and assist them into our flimsy print gowns with the gap in the back.

Many arrive with an entourage and relatives make fast friends with each other and with our staff. Sleep is snatched in recliners, ethnic dinners are concocted in the microwave and hours are whiled away in conversation. Tips for surviving this immigration camp are exchanged.

Days are filled with tests or awaiting procedures, such as CT scans, X-rays, myelograms, angiograms, biopsies, laminectomies — and dozens of other procedures. Technicians turned detectives extract evidence from blood, urine, sputum and stool. Dieticians, respiratory therapists, occupational therapists require patient time as well.

As nightfall approaches, the flurry of activities is diminished. The busy hospital routine slows and is no longer a defense against the terrors of the night. No amount of money, no unlimited beauty, no special privilege, no position can protect our patients now as they dread the lonely trek toward dawn. As nurses we offer a back rub, a face washing, tooth brushing, knowing our presence will provide a captive ear. Before the lights are dimmed patients try out their tentative philosophies, hoping for confirmation and courage.

"I've always tried to help others. The Lord will get me through this."

"I always wanted control. I was hard on my kids. Do you think that's why I got this tumor?"

"I always wanted to be governor, but as an honest man I can't make it."

"What's important now is time with my family. I wish I'd known that 30 years ago."

"It's just stress. I'll sell my business and relax."

"My mother is coming tomorrow. I'll be all right once she gets here."

"My husband takes such wonderful care of me. He's such a good man. He doesn't deserve this."

"I won't go to a nursing home. I'd rather just die."

"I'm afraid I won't wake up from surgery. I have a bad feeling about it. And my feelings usually steer me right."

"I was so happy. Then my whole life changed in just a half hour."

"I am so tired. I am ready to die, but it's so hard to leave them."

Standing in the doorway of a darkened room, I think these patients are like the ill-fated pasengers on the Titanic. It was all such fun. The people. The costumes. The games. The music. The diversion. But the party is over now. The iceberg of mortality has been hit. The vessel is no longer seaworthy. Modern medicine launches its lifeboats; some will climb aboard, consenting to medical treatment, knowing the ride will be wild and the waves overwhelming. There is room for many but not all. There is pride but also uncertainty in setting ashore those who are healed and who will enjoy a temporary unfathomable sea that awaits what each of us must face in time.

Joyce Nelson, RN
Rochester, MN

I AM A NURSE

As I dressed for work on Nurses' Day, I left the business suit in the closet and donned my uniform, complete with cap. I thought today my statement is simple. Above everything else that I represent, I am a nurse!

Reflecting over 20 years of nursing (where did the time go?), it's very difficult to single out just one patient that changed my life. The faces of many patients float through my mind . . . some of them bring a smile to my lips, while others bring tears to my eyes, and still others bring thoughts of anger because I was unable to save them or help them.

Can I ever forget the panic that occurred when no doctor was available and I delivered that baby . . . the exhilarating feeling that came when that little being let out that first cry . . . and, oh, the look of awe on the mother's face when she first held her child?

NURSE

Can I forget the late night rounds when I found a young wife and mother crying because her pathology report came back positive for breast cancer or the feeling of total inadequacy as I sat there and let her express her anger, fear, frustration and loss? I stayed with her until she dropped off to sleep. As I left the room, I thought "Why?"

Can I ever forget the inner peace that I felt when I saw death occur for that elderly patient or cancer patient who had worked through the death process? I held their hands and talked to them until life processes had ceased.

Nursing is so many things to each of us. I would like to think I have made a difference. For me, if I make one person smile and feel like someone cares for them, then my day has been a good one.

Finally, the patient that I remember most. She and her husband had been married many years. They had not been blessed with children. Over the course of six months, she watched me swell with the impending birth of my child. I, in turn, watched her wither as the cancer ravaged her body. We became very close. I would spend my extra time in her room letting her talk abot her life, her happiness with her husband, and her disappointments. Near the end, she gave me the greatest compliment of all. She said "If I had ever had a daughter, I would have wanted her to be a nurse like you. I couldn't have stood this if you hadn't been with me."

Through my years of nursing, I have thought of her words often and have tried to hold onto the qualities that she found in me as a young nurse.

Sharon Teixeira, RN, CNA
Kailua-Kona, Hawaii

Reprinted by special permission from "Riverside Nurse," Riverside Health System, Newport News, Virginia.

THE LITTLE THINGS

Janet was a beautiful and energetic young woman before becoming a patient in our intensive care unit. Her previous lifestyle was painfully obvious by the clues on her bulletin board. There were so many cards we couldn't keep them all up at the same time. Pictures of her family and college classmates framed the lower left corner of the bulletin board. That one picture of Janet with her three best friends made it impossible for us to ignore the harsh reality of how much her life had changed in the past two months.

Janet had been complaining of general malaise and aching joints just prior to her hospitalization. When medication and rest did not alleviate the symptoms and they began to get worse, her mother took her to the hospital for evaluation. Because her neurological exam was not completely normal, she was admitted for further evaluation.

A week on general medical floor left the physicians puzzled and Janet's symptoms began to worsen: decreased level of consciousness, painful joints, edema, abnormal laboratory results, and some difficulty with respiration appeared. Finally, one afternoon when her mother was present, Janet's respiratory status and neurological status decompensated so rapidly that endotracheal intubation and a stat transfer to our intensive care unit was necessary.

When I admitted Janet to intensive care unit that afternoon she was edematous (swollen with excess accumulation of fluid in the body), and having trouble with the respirator. Sedation was necessary to prepare her for yet another CT scan which ultimately revealed nothing. For me, this was a particularly heart-wrenching experience from the very start. We do not have a pediatric service at our hospital, so taking care of a nineteen-year-old woman was a new experience for me. In addition to attending to her serious physical problems, we had to assist the emotional needs of her family, especially her mother, who was desperately worried and in need of considerable support.

Day after day Janet's mom and her aunt would sit by the bedside watching her condition continue to deteriorate. Over the course of a few weeks Janet became completely unresponsive, listless and developed problems necessitating several chest tubes and eventually high frequency jet ventilation just to maintain her PO^2 in the sixties.

(Ed.: The immediately preceding means that the staff was trying to maintain the patient's oxygen level at sixty or more mm. of mercury. A healthy, young person might measure 95 mm. while the level in an older person would drop. Some experts say the average might run between 80 and 90 or perhaps 100, many factors affecting the statistic.)

To both the nursing and medical staff it slowly became obvious that Janet was not going to make it. Her unknown disease was taking away her beautiful young life bit by bit day by day. It was particularly painful to watch her mother and aunt talk to her by the hour and continue to question us and build hope on the infrequent, spastic twitches of her swollen body.

There was not one inch of her body that was left untouched by the sometimes useless wonders of modern critical care medicine. Invasive monitoring and intravenous lines cluttered and bruised her arms and neck. Several chest tubes were crowded into different areas of her thorax. Her groins were scarred and bandaged from blood drawing and central lines. But the most disturbing thing for her family to look at was her face. She had always prided herself on her impeccable grooming but now half of her head was shaved with an intracranial pressure monitor jutting out the side, her lips were scabbed, sputum drained from her mouth and nose, and what seemed like several rolls of tape were necessary to anchor the tubes in place.

Soon after Janet was admitted into our unit, I began to wash and French braid her hair every day. I realized that our expert nursing care was not going to save her, or even protect the integrity of her body. As a nurse I needed something to offer the family as well as to help me feel just a little better than totally useless every time I walked into the room. I also believe that ICU nurses who deal with high technology and critically ill patients every day find it is important not to forget the caring, non-technical, humanistic parts of nursing. After all, those are the fundamental values upon which the modern profession of nursing is built.

After six painful weeks in our intensive care unit, Janet died. It was very difficult for her family as well as for the medical and nursing staff. Perhaps the worst part for everyone was that even her autopsy did not confirm the exact cause of her death. That is something we will all have to live with. However, several weeks after she died I received a card and note from her mome, which read "God bless you, Karen. Thank you for doing Janet's hair."

The card instantly filled me with incredible emotion. It helped me once again to realize that sometimes it is the little things that mean the most. There is so much comfort in simply caring for those in pain, even when all else fails. As an ICU nurse I hope I never forget that.

Karen K. Giuliano, RN, MS, CCRN
Palmyra, Virginia

FORMER ARMY NURSE HAS MANY MEMENTOS

With a strong feeling of patriotism and what might have been a foretaste of today's women's liberation movement—Mrs. Marcella Selbert "felt I should be in service" says her daughter.

As a result, Mrs. Carl F. Kantola—then Miss Helen Selbert, R.N., has a collection of souvenirs from her days as an Army nurse during World War II.

They include a pencil portrait of herself by an Italian artist and a German Iron Cross presented by an Italian physician, both of whom were prisoners of war. She also has a heavy silver and coral bracelet and ring from Casablanca given to her by the captain who commanded the POW camp and whom she dated.

But most precious to the Rochester, NY, native who served in French North Africa and later Italy, is a collection of news clippings—especially one written by an Air Corps corporal who was her patient. In it he wrote, in part:

"IF EVER MEDALS were given for meritorious service beyond the call of duty, then one of your local girls—a pretty, red-haired miss—deserved one. I am referring to 2nd Lt. Helen E. Selbert, our charming Army nurse.

NURSE

"She is possessed of the nicest voice that a wounded soldier ever listened to. Each night just after medication time when the lights are turned low, Lt. Selbert is sure to be there in our ward singing request numbers for these injured heroes. To hear her sing the 'Ave Maria' and many other classical and semi-classical numbers each night at this time is the greatest pleasure these boys know.

"I have seen men restless and jittery from the effects of battle slip off into slumber that medicine would not give them when Lt. Selbert sends her silvery voice softly winging down the hospital aisles."

The corporal, D. B. Crimmings, sent the article to Lt. Selbert's hometown paper without her knowledge, and she didn't know of it until her mother gave her a framed copy when she came home in 1945.

Mrs. Kantola, who said she had been singing "as long as I can remember", added that she "sang all through St. Mary's hospital in Rochester" where she was graduated before going on to the staff of Strong Memorial hospital there and later to Columbia Presbyterian hospital, New York, as a neurological nurse.

She studied one summer at the Eastman School of Music at Rochester and sang with Guy Fraser Harrison's civic chorus. Her voice graced political and other dinners when the Kantolas lived in Dumont where Kantola was a councilman.

Mrs. Kantola spent approximately three years in service, serving as medical-surgical and later as psychiatric nurse with the 43rd station hospital in French North Africa and later the 114th station hospital near Naples and Rome.

SHE HAS MEMORIES full store:

* Of living and nursing in tents in Africa—racing to put wet cloths over the faces of patients so they could breathe when sand siroccos struck.

* And of the time an Arab sheik offered her commanding colonel "two camels plus some territory" to add "the girl with the sunburst hair" to his harem.

* Of the open-top showers in Italy and the attraction they had for low-swooping Air Force pilots.

"When we complained to the colonel he told us next time it happened to get the plane's number," she recalls with a trace of indignation.

* Of the night the hospital in Africa received 500 malaria patients all at once. And of the time they were bombed five nights straight in Naples.

"We were supposed to run from the fifth floor to the basement," she said. "The first night I did. After that I pulled the sheet over my head and told the nurses (under her command) they could go. You could have broken your neck going down all those stairs."

* And there was the night she stood far in the back with the troops at Bob Hope's 1945 Christmas show, only to have him spot her. (He must have eyes like telescopes," she said.) "And tell her to come down here in front, you beautiful angel."

When Hope appeared at the Garden State Arts Center two years ago the Kantolas were in the audience. She went backstage to see him and "We hugged and kissed each other," she said.

Mrs. Kantola met her husband after the war through his niece, a nurse with whom she had served. He's a mechanical and electrical engineer who retired in 1967 after 47 years with the New York Central Railroad where he earned 12 patents.

Among those he considers the most important was a patent for a method of streamlining a steam engine that was applied to the Commodore Vanderbilt and one for an improved water scoop that enabled steam engines to take on water while travelling at speeds up to 85 mphs.

Sandra Otto Cummings
Asbury Park, NJ

Reprinted by special permission from the Asbury Park Press, Neptune, NJ, June 15, 1980 issue.

NO, NOT NOW

They stood up one-by-one. It looked like "The Wave", the cheer that crowds do at ball games. Two rows of them. I caught the movement out of the corner of my eye. This is peculiar behavior, I thought, for people attending a concert.

It was no cheer. It was an alarm.

"Is there a doctor here?" "Someone call 911."

I didn't think. I just moved. Somehow I crossed the laps of five people and found myself calling for people to stand back. Fortunately, some big bruisers had come to the rescue and were carrying a very large man from his seat by the wall to the aisle.

I was on him in a split second. Someone was checking his pulse and beginning cardiac compressions. I began mouth-to-mouth ventilations.

We got him back.

"Watch him. He'll go again." I knew the advice was sound, my memory racing back to resuscitations in the past.

He did go again. This time I was on compressions. Someone else was ventilating him. When I looked up, the paramedics were racing up the stairs.

As I replaced another, I stumbled back to allow the rescuer into the narrow aisle., An arm caught me and it was then I started shaking. A police officer sat me down and asked me for my name and address. As I answered his questions, I made the transition from CPR rescuer to bystander-observer. I noted with awe the adept handling of the situation by the paramedics.

It was with great relief that I watched the paramedics carry away our patient on a stretcher. He was breathing on his own; his heart beat had resumed and he was conscious. As his wife passed me in the aisle I reached out to her and gave her arm a squeeze.

The value of proficiency in CPR was never more dear to me than it was that evening. The concert started forty-five minutes late. The whole situation had an unreal quality to it. Minutes before I was part of an effort that said "No, not now" to death. Then, minutes later, I was listening to a favorite performer sing some favorite songs. But as I sat there, I kept thinking of that corny closing to a CPR film I had seen—"Another heart too good to die."

Kathleen Beyerman, RN, EdD
Winchester, Massachusetts

VIETNAM MEMORIES

"We served in Vietnam at about the same time and I guess I never had or took the opportunity to thank one of the nurses who served over there at the critical time, so I will take the opportunity to do so now."

The letter was signed by a total stranger, dated March, 1990, 22 years after I returned to what we called "the world." My reply tried to match his elegance: "Thank you very much for your gracious note. Would that I could share its beautiful message with all of my sisters and brothers with whom I served."

About 8,000 nurses, approximately 85% of whom were women, served in the military or as civilian nurses and I can safely say virtually none of us expected a thank you. This was not the first time a fellow vet has asked me to accept his gratitude on behalf of all nurses but each time it happens I feel somewhat perplexed, a little uncomfortable because, like him, I was just doing my job. But my heart glows with a special warmth and appreciation for each person who cares enough to express that sentiment decades after the war.

The same day that letter arrived, a coincidence happened that, if I were writing fiction, would be cut by the editor as being just unbelievable. The telephone rang in my law office and the voice said "Hi, I'm calling from D.C. I work for the government out here. I know you were a nurse in 'Nam and I just wanted to talk. You see, I lost my legs there in October, 1970, and I just now got up enough courage, or whatever, to wheel over to the Wall for the first time. And, you know what? I found my name on the Wall." He'd been busy trying to find out why he had been included on the list of those who had died in Vietnam.

We talked for quite a while: he especially wanted to talk about when he had been wounded and brought into a hospital near Da Nang, not far from the demilitarized zone (DMZ) between North and South Vietnam. The triage nurse injected him with morphine, which didn't touch his pain and he kept asking for more. She said "No, I can't do it. You've had a huge amount; you have to wait another three hours." A tourniquet had stopped the bleeding from his left leg which had been torn off above the ankle, but his right leg continued to ooze, and his pain intensified. He kept begging her for more morphine. She said she'd check with the doctor and a few minutes later returned with a little red football-shaped capsule and told him that he could have this pill even though he couldn't have any more morphine. She sat down with him, talked for awhile, kept reassuring him he'd be all right and not to worry. He said "I relaxed, listened, and in a half hour or so, the pill worked, the pain disappeared, I stopped worrying and went to sleep.

When I got back to the states and I needed a stool softener, a nurse gave me Colace*—the same little red pill I'd been given in triage! I've believed in placebos ever since, and I especially believe in nurses."

As my middle years continue to distance me from my youth, these experiences with my fellow vets do much to keep me in touch with memories that were made in Vietnam. The patients, the colleagues, the friends emerge from the depths, sometimes missing important pieces—names without faces, faces without names. My pride in serving my country during those difficult times is renewed, as are my negative feelings about the war in which I served.

I was 24 when my Boeing 707 touched down at Bien Hoa airport, 17 miles northeast of Saigon, 13,000 miles away from home. There were 60 of us army nurses, men and women, who struggled down the steep steps through the oven-like heat of a sunny day in South Vietnam. A grenade-proof bus, with windows painted army green and thick screens wrapped around the outside, drove us to the 90th Replacement Battalion, about five miles away in Long Binh.

Long Binh had been carved out of the jungle, defoliated and covered in laterite, a reddish soil well remembered for the ease with which it clung to clothes, eyes, nose, and so forth. At Long Binh we received our assignments, about a third of us going to the 36th Evacuation hospital in Vung Tau, 45 miles southeast of Saigon, at the tip of a ten mile long peninsula.

Vung Tau was the antithesis of the sprawling army base at Long Binh. The peninsula had been developed by the French before the turn of the century as a resort town. Villas and hotels were everywhere, restaurants sold food prepared for French gourmets—a variety of white fish, lobster, poultry and pork, as well as fresh fruit, bananas, pineapples and vegetables.

The 36th didn't have any housing for the staff on the army base, so we lived in a three-story hotel a couple of miles away and often ate on "the economy" instead of at the hospital. One of the many

---

*Colace—Registered product name of Mead Johnson & Company.

puzzles in Vung Tau was why we were never shelled, never attacked. Why, much to our ongoing astonishment, did Viet Cong walk the streets, shopping and dining unmolested. After all these years I've still only been able to trace down that Vung Tau had been a safe haven for troops from both sides for as long as anyone could remember. Apparently this was an unwritten understanding by parties unknown throughout the decades of the various conflicts in which Vietnam had been engaged.

But, not having that perspective in 1967, the staff of the 36th worried that our peace would end momentarily, that instead of only caring for victims of war, we, too, would be injured. My favorite form of repressing these anxieties was reading, which also helped me escape the stress of caring for the wounded, most of whom were only 19 years old. I had come to Vietnam with a specialty in caring for critically ill adults but I was not emotionally prepared to find myself on my first day assigned to give nursing care to ten severely wounded 18 and 19 year olds and two equally sick Vietnamese solders, who were both 16.

During my three months on that intensive care unit my memories began to form and friendships grew.

One of the women with whom I had flown over had become actively involved, in off-duty time, in helping build a clinic for dependents of men stationed at the Vietnamese military school in Vung Tau. Her boundless energy was directed at sending letters to everyone she'd ever met, asking for supplies and equipment. Mail was super slow in Vietnam and highly frustrating on a good day, but she never stopped mailing her requests. To this day I can still see her freckled face beaming as supplies came in the mail, often only one instrument at a time. She organized the rest of us to attend the clinic when it was finally opened, to check teeth and to dispense pills, soap and good will. Although the army hoped such activity would win the hearts and minds of the peasants, we saw only an opportunity to help our hosts cope with disease and poverty.

At the 36th the ICU staff took turns being on call for the emergency room to triage the casualties. A few weeks after I arrived, my corpsman and I were summoned to the E.R. The Dustoffs (Huey helicopters, whose nickname was also their official radio call sign) had already landed as we ran through the door of the Quonset hut which functioned as the E.R. I ran to the first gurney and to this day can still see the man's face, his brown eyes fixed open, the back of his neck and head blown away. I rushed to the next man and can still hear the relief in his voice as he said "Hello, sister." My hands shook as I wrapped a blood pressure cuff around his arm and fought down the nausea as I tried to make some coherent reply while I gazed at the bloody stumps of his legs and realized that he was Australian, as were the other 11 who came in that afternoon.

My memory does not tell me whether I cared for those three after they came out of surgery, but there are many other patients whom I remember well.

One of these was Bill, a 19 year old mechanic from St. Louis. While he and his sergeant had been stranded on a lonely jungle road and Bill was fixing their stalled jeep, Viet Cong gunned down the sergeant and threw a grenade under the open hood. Bill lost both his arms just above the elbows.

I had been working in recovery room when he came out of the operating room. When I took his blood pressure he opened his eyes, looked first at one stump, suspended on an IV pole, then at me. I could hear the question in his big brown eyes, but I couldn't think of anything to say. Tears started rolling down his cheeks. I bent over and hugged him, swallowing the tears I knew I shouldn't show him.

During the next few days Bill made a remarkable attempt to cope with his tragedy. He talked about his loss, how he was going to have to learn to be something other than a mechanic, although maybe with the right artificial limbs he could go back to that work. As he went from bed to bed, he pushed around his IV stand and talked with the guys who were awake. When Bill left for Toyko all of our names and addresses were tucked in his pocket, but to my knowledge no one ever heard of him again.

Another one of my special memories is about Randy Brown—not his real name. He, too, was only 19. I first took care of him shortly after I was assigned to be head nurse on ward three. I had resisted that assignment explaining to our chief nurse that I had never had any experience nor training to be one. Despite that fact and that I was only a very green first lieutenant, she whisked away my protest, saying that I was the highest ranking officer in the hospital who wasn't already a head nurse, and that army protocol required that I take the position.

Randy said he was a Tennessee plowboy and he looked the part—tall, tan, lean and strong. He had big blue eyes, a bright smile, and a habit of rubbing a leather medallion he had hanging with his dog tags. The first time he was hurt was when his buddy, unloading a truck, had dropped a Claymore mine, which exploded, killing himself and several other young soldiers. But Randy was fortunate. A dozen of the sharp metal arrows from the mine had torn open the flesh of his left leg but none had permanently damaged any muscle. After the surgeon had removed the metal and had sutured his wounds it was necessary for him to be treated for a couple of weeks with antibiotics and a pain medication before he could return to fighting.

He spent those weeks in my ward three, recuperating, gradually regaining full strength in his leg, exercising and spending time on the ward master's work detail. He would run errands, answer my phone, empty wastebaskets, and make himself useful around the ward, all the while doing Abbott and Costello routines with the medical corpsmen.

The last Saturday he was there I had to work the evening shift, missing out on a party with my housemates. I decided that ward three should have its own party. Randy eagerly volunteered to pick up the beer and snacks I ordered from the PX. After the evening treatments were done and the medications passed out, we played some rock and roll on a borrowed record player and had our party. The medical corpsmen thought I was crazy and the stuffy old ward master was furious but we had a quiet, safe time away from the war.

That Monday Randy went back to his unit. He came back in May with a wound more severe and disfiguring than those of March. His platoon had been ambushed on night patrol and he had been shot. The bullet had ripped up his left arm, cutting a wide path through his flesh from his elbow to his shoulder. But the surgeons were able to find enough tissue to sew back together without impairing the arm's functioning. He was healthy and well fed and recovered rapidly.

He was as helpful as before, as pleasant, and spent even more of his time taking care of the patients whose injuries were worse than his. He read to them, wrote their letters, fetched water for them, pushed them around in their wheelchairs—this time doing Crosby and Hope jokes.

After a couple of weeks he knew he was going back to his unit on Monday. He asked if we were going to have another party on Saturday, like before. I said "Of course." Again we had a very nice, safe party, away from the war. One of the corpsmen, Joey, brought his guitar. Randy organized the refreshments and served everybody. Those patients well enough to get out of bed gathered around those who could not and we sang songs until 11 o'clock. Randy, the corpsmen and I tucked everyone in for the night. The night nurse came on duty to find everyone asleep or resting quietly.

That Monday Randy went back to his unit. He was again full of health and vitality. He came in July to see several of his buddies who had been wounded. He brought them a radio, some cigarettes and candy. He visited with everyone, even the guys he didn't know, smiling sunshine all the while, his healthy blue eyes sparkling their warmth. As he left he said "Goodbye, Miss Boulay. If you ever get to Tennessee, y'all come see us, ya hear?" "Sure, Randy" and he was gone back to his unit.

Shortly thereafter I was transferred to another hospital to work in their intensive care unit. Only the very sick and badly wounded young soldiers were cared for in that ward.

Although these patients never returned to the fighting once they left us, we rarely had anyone die while in our ward. This was primarily because of the medical treatment they received within minutes of the devastating trauma they suffered in the fighting. Thus many young soliders survived injuries that otherwise would have killed them quickly. The lifesaving surgery would be done, the infection staved off with massive doses of antibiotics, the body allowed to regain stability and, in three or four days, the grievously compromised young life would be sent to Tokyo or to the states for long-term care or perhaps death. Many we cared for died after leaving us.

The infamous Tet offensive began at 3 A.M. on January 31, 1968. It was the first time the hospital staff had experienced being smack in the middle of the fighting. The ammunition dump a mile down the road was blown up, caving in one wall of our ward. We could hear gunfire almost continuously. Snipers were shooting at soldiers standing in lines outside a neighboring supply unit. We had to wear helmets, sleep in bunkers sometimes and work twelve-hour shifts.

I was working the 7 P.M. to 7 A.M. shift in mid-February. The early days of the offensive had passed. The badly mangled marines from our embassy in Saigon, which had been overrun, had been cared for and sent on to Tokyo. We were trying not to accept too many casualties for a few hours because the huge army division down the road was gearing up for some intense fighting and large numbers of severly wounded soldiers would be coming in. Therefore, the ICU was quiet when I came on duty that February evening.

The day nurse and I sat down at the desk. She said she had only one patient in my section of the ward but he was in unusually bad shape. His unit had been attacked and he had been hit by several automatic rifle bullets which had shattered most of his lungs and intestines. Grenade fragments had lodged in his liver and pancreas and the surgeons were unable to remove them. One kidney was gone and the other one was shutting down. He had been unconscious since he had come out of surgery. He was too unstable to send on to Tokyo . . . and she doubted this 20-year-old youngster would make it through the night. As I got up to go see him, I looked for his name on the chart.

Randy Brown.

I rushed to the bedside. His skin was sickly yellow; he was barely breathing; and what urine was in the containers was brown. He felt hot and dry and his pulse was weak. I picked up his hand and just stared at him. He was almost unrecognizable but he was Randy Brown indeed.

"Randy," I whispered, "Oh, Randy." It was like discovering one of my own children lying in my intensive care unit. I took his temperature — it was 105 degrees. His blood pressure — inaudible. I kept talking to him.

"Randy, this is Miss Boulay. Wake up. Wake up, please."

I gave him his medication and rubbed his neck.

"Randy." He was still breathing. I kept on talking.

"Randy." I changed his bandages. He was bleedly profusely from the massive wound in his abdomen and from where his kidney had been.

"Randy."

"Hi, Miss Boulay." He heard me!

We talked slowly, softly, no jokes, no smiles. He wondered where his leather medallion was. I held his hand. His eyes were sunken, gray and yellow.

About midnight he closed those eyes, his breathing shallow. We stopped talking while I continued to hold his hand. Soon Randy Brown, his sparkle gone, died. Then I cried.

In early March I returned to the world. Afraid that the sadness and hurt that erupted once my plane touched down at Travis Air Force base in California had changed me in some unacceptable way, I kept myself from going home to my east coast family for six months. When I did find the courage to go home, I was welcomed with all the love and hugs I had so badly needed when I had first stepped off that plane.

D. M. Boulay, RN, JD
Minneapolis, MN

CARRIE WANTED TO MAKE SON'S WEDDING

All Carrie, age 57, wanted was to be home. Everyone to whom she talked said that was impossible.

I met her four months after she was diagnosed as having metastatic cancer in all her bones. American doctors gave her no hope so she had gone to Mexico, hoping for a cure there. After two months of treatment there she had collapsed and had been transferred to a hospital in my community.

My first meeting with Carrie in my hospital found her with casts on all limbs and bald from chemotherapy. She would do anything to go home but the health professionals said she was too weak and would break more bones, that her family couldn't care for her. In the hospital it took five people just to put her on the bedpan.

She wanted to go home because a son was getting married and she wanted to be there.

I asked the rehab staff to start training the family to move her around. People in her church also volunteered so they were trained too. Carrie's social worker was able to get her eligible for Medicaid home care benefits, so six weeks after we started, and longer than she was expected to live, Carrie went home.

But that was just the beginning.

Keeping her home was even more difficult. Her blood count dropped. Her doctors insisted she should return to the hospital for more chemotherapy. Medicaid wouldn't pay for more nurses, so I taught her youngest son to give injections. I drew her blood weekly for the lab. I trained one of the church women and hired her to care for Carrie for forty hours a week, paid by Medicaid, relieving Josh, her husband, from much of her care.

Carrie began to think she would live long enough to see her son get married in three months. Repeatedly I had to tell her physicians she couldn't be hospitalized because she was intimidated by them and would start crying at the mere thought of returning.

The worst time was two days before the wedding when Carrie spiked a temperature of 104 degrees and called her doctor for relief; I understand that he told her she would die immediately if she didn't return to the hospital. She called me, crying. All she wanted to do was to stay alive to go to the wedding. I called the doctor and said "I'm terribly sorry but Carrie can't come to the hospital. She has to be in her son's wedding this weekend. She could come for treatment on Monday." The doctor indicated that she'd probably be dead by then, to which I answered "At least she would have been in this wedding which means so much to her."

Family and friends took turns sponging her to break the fever. At one point I had them wrap her completely in wet sheets, even her casts. Her fever broke.

Carrie never looked more radiant than she did at the wedding. We curled her wig, dressed her in a red and black dress with a big floppy, red hat and around her shoulder we threw a feathered boa. Her husband wore a tux. Two physical therapists and I placed her on a stretcher which could be folded into a wheelchair so she could sit up or lie down if she tired. I inserted a catheter so she wouldn't need a bedpan, hiding the bag beneath her dress.

The wedding ceremony was beautiful and the phtographers took hundreds of family pictures. Carrie not only made her son's wedding but she celebrated her 37th wedding anniversary two months later. She also had a chance to make an inspirational tape for her church. At her memorial service her husband thanked me publicly for giving them thirteen months at home with Carrie. I was only doing what she wanted done.

Dee Billops, RN
Albuquerque, NM

THE NURSE

I am not an angel of mercy
Or a handmaiden, who with a doctor flirts.
I was educated, not trained, for my profession.
I am an advocate, a healer, a professional nurse.
My hands have touched the soft newborn
And caressed the sore limbs of the dying.
Such experiences do not make me immune to death;
I, too, have feelings and have walked away crying.
Chronic shortages of needed equipment and qualified personnel
Frustrate me, and I want to quit in despair.
But still I press on, and do my best
To give my patients the best of my care.

Rita A. Jablonski, RN
Philadelphia, PA

Reprinted with permission of the Philadelphia, PA Daily News.

THE FIRST GOODBYE

He was my first primary patient. I had just passed my nursing boards and started my first job as an RN. Curt became a very special patient to me. He had pancreatic cancer with a poor prognosis and had come to our hospital for a pancreatectomy (removal of the pancreas). When Curt arrived on the floor post-op I'm not sure who was feeling worse—he or I. I felt overwhelmed with the tubes, drains and pumps and had a hard time "seeing" through them to the patient. As I overcame my fears, I came to realize my full potential as a primary nurse.

Curt had a great family. His wife, children and grandchildren spent a great deal of time with him and we got to know each other well. The Christmas holiday came, but he still wasn't feeling any better. Fortunately, that didn't stop a celebration. There was a tree, gifts and lots of laughter. Unfortunately, Curt didn't improve and continued to weaken. At each medical crisis we were able to pull him through and to buy him time. It took me some time to realize finally that Curt was never going to get better and that time was all we could actually give him.

Finally the issue of DNR came up. (Ed.: DNR means to give "Do Not Resuscitate" instructions—i.e., do not attempt to revive at apparent death. Obviously given only in severe cases when authorities and family agree to let the terminal patient die.)

I realized this DNR decision was one of the hardest with which I would have to deal. After several days of discussion, Curt and his family changed his status to DNR. It was the realization of a type of defeat. We, the health care team, with advanced technology on our side, were unable to cure Curt. Emotional support became the final and most important intervention. My nursing goal at this point was to help Curt and his family cope with the final stages of death and dying.

As his primary nurse I felt it was important to discuss where he wanted to die. His family wanted him to be at home, but Curt was reluctant to go, and even more reluctant to discuss his reasons. Finally his wife came to me and asked if I could find out why he didn't want to go tome. It was while I was helping him wash that morning that I broached the subject. Curt looked at me with tears in his eyes, then explained. "I don't want my family to think of the home in which so much happiness occurred and the bedroom where I've spent the last forty years of my life with my wife, as the place where I died, where sadness occurred. I also don't want my wife to have to deal with my body after I die."

I think Curt felt relief after talking about this and was more at peace.

When his wife came that afternoon we discussed his answers and she suggested that maybe he would, at least, like to come home for a day. Curt agreed. Through the help of other staff members, Curt was able to go home on a leave of absence, three days later. I was not there to see him go, but I worked the night he came back. He was very tired and looked more jaundiced and was weaker. Instinctively I knew he would not make it through the night. He fell asleep around eleven PM and at four AM woke up briefly and smiled; then he said his last goodbye. He fell asleep while I sat with him. As the dawn broke, Curt took his last breath.

I said my first goodbye.

Stacey Smith, RN
Waltham, Massachusetts

HOW COULD I COUNSEL HER?

I was an RN in the operating room in 1972 when abortions were legalized. I was exempt from doing Terminations of Pregnancies because of my religious convictions. At the time I knew of a few close relatives who were having abortions every couple of months, so my religious convictions were no more.

Two years later at the age of 42 I had a baby. When she was two weeks old I was called in for an emergency in the operating room. The patient was being forced by her husband to have an abortion. She was 42 years old, like me, and pleaded with me to tell her she was doing the right thing.

What a spot for me to be in. Can you imagine how hard it was for me to convince a woman my own age, just before she was going under anesthesia, that she was justified in what she was doing? And here I had just been delivered of my own baby, and me with a problem of religious convictions!

An unidentified RN
Long Island, NY

HE SHOULD HAVE BEEN A NURSE

As a young boy he wanted to be a physician which, to him, meant being a surgeon but, alas, that was not to be. Polio in the younger years wiped out the flexibility of his right hand and wrist and it was obvious he would never have the dexterity to be a surgeon. But the sad part is that little town didn't have a counselor to direct him toward some other kind of medicine, or nursing. In either profession he would have been happy and made the contribution he pictured coming from being a surgeon. So medicine and nursing lost a good prospect.

He should have been a nurse. It was long apparent that he had a natural affinity for caring for, stroking, a person needing help. As an older man, his wife was laying in bed coughing her head off from a winter cold of unknown causes. She's a strong-willed Minnesotan and prefers to stick it out rather than use an OTC (over-the-counter) product, much less pay a physician thirty dollars for a prescription for an antibiotic, which probably wouldn't help her any more than it did her husband. So she thinks.

He preferred his dear departed mother's technique and insisted on applying a little Vick's VapoRub* in the external hollow of her throat and wrap the neck with a long flannel cloth—actually cotton stocking material left over from a hospital trip. Within ten minutes she quit coughing and was sleeping soundly. Sometimes the old wives' procedures work well.

A real RN or an MD would have used much better procedures and products but I also believe they'd agree that we should take some mild steps ourselves.

Anyway, I was that boy and man.

William H. Hull, MA
Edina, MN

---

*© Richardson-Vicks, Inc.

THE GIFT OF LOVE AND UNDERSTANDING

(An interview with a loving, sensitive nurse who just happens to be blind.)

What is your role with a cardiac patient? What do you do?

Primarily, I get the patient ready for discharge . . . to face life after being in the hospital. To face life after what he has gone through here.

You must have a lot of psychology or psychiatric training?

I like doing this because I have a critical care background and also a lot of group therapy background. I feel that is just as important as taking the correct medication. You can't have one without the other.

I'll bet a lot of people are very pleased with what you do for them — to help set their goals, to keep them alive, to learn to live with this new problem.

This is a great place to be — here in the Cardiac Special Care unit for two days, four days, seven days after cardiac bypass, heart attack or whatever. And then we don't want to just tell them goodbye — you're now on your own. It's not so easy to be in their shoes. It's difficult for them to make changes after having been around for 25 years, or 75 years. It's a big part of my job — cardiac aftercare, meaning contact and care for the patient even after he has gone home.

Is that what "Cardiac Case Care" means — which I see on your name tag?

Case care is the cardiac umbrella term. I have contact with the patient before surgery, before angiograms, before any procedure, before they even come into the hospital. I keep them informed of their upcoming procedure, answer any questions, help them anticipate what they may want to bring to the hospital.

Frequently I see people coming into the hospital for special tests and sometimes I can alleviate their worry by telling them "Look, this is

94

not a painful procedure. I've had it." I can see where your contact would be of great relief to them.

Scans and all the procedures are totally new to people. This person needs this information, reassurance, even guidance.

You could perform much beyond cardiac service.

I'd probably like it to be, but this is a first step.

When you go into a patient's room and he sees your name tag which says "Shelli Nicoson, RN"—he says to himself "This must be a blind nurse. She's got a white cane and a dog. What's going on here?"

They don't hear anything I say during the first few minutes I'm here. They're busy looking at me, wondering how much I can see, how I lost my sight, how in the world I'm going to help them when I can't see. When they hear that I am a nurse, the whole thing starts over again. I've learned to sit down and let them meld through me a little bit to understand. It's a process, but that's okay. I'd probably feel the same way.

I bet there are many times when you feel your first interview is almost wasted.

Sometimes after the first five minutes I'll say "Do you remember my name? Do you know what I do?" And they usually don't. Sometimes on the phone I'll ask that same question and when they hesitate I'll say "I'm the blind nurse." Then they remember immediately.

It's not something that I want people to remember me by—that I'm a blind nurse—but it does help identify me. I wouldn't want to be the subject of a book called "Blind Nurse" because there is too much more to my life than only that.

As you said to me the other day: I just lost my sight. I didn't lose my mind.

Yes, or any other part of me.

When you go into a patient's room for the first time, are you expecting a rebuff?

Yes, that says it exactly, but I try to go in and not be defensive.

NURSE

There have been a couple of times when I was verbally assaulted.

One time this last week I went into a patient's room — a man who had been diabetic for thirty-five years, was on dialysis, and a lot of stuff. I went to talk about what I was going to do for him but he wasn't ready to hear anything from me.

Right away he said "Now what do you want. Yeah, I can see you have a white cane but what does that mean?" I said "The white cane has nothing to do with why I'm here." He then retorted "I don't want to hear any of your problems, I've got enough of my own."

I had to stop and say to myself that he's not mad at me; he doesn't even know me, so I told him that. "I know you're not really angry at me. Something else must be upsetting you and I'm sorry." I know that he was worried about life and death, depressed over the way his health had been deteriorating. The man has reason to be angry at the world.

How about the other nurses? I have seen one who helps steer you around once in a while, sort of protectionism from her to you. She's really a close friend.

Bill, you know who that is! You're right on. She's not a nurse, though. That's my mom. (Laughter)

The nurses and I have a good time because I let them know that it's okay to joke about it. Sometimes it can be funny. When I first came here everybody was apprehensive. They didn't know what I needed or didn't need. They didn't know how to handle such expressions as "You should see that" or "Look over here." I use those expressions myself. I say "Gosh, it's good to see you again" or "I haven't seen you for quite a while" and everybody knows I don't really mean "see" as in vision. It's great that we've learned to laugh about it and it's worked out well. I have many very close friends here.

I know that I'm blind and it's okay to make jokes about it. We all laugh about it.

I can see where you are an extension of the nurses' self. They must truly appreciate what you are doing — which saves them time. And we know that the nurse constantly fights for better use of her time.

All of the surgery procedures and other things that are going to happen on this unit, I know about. Whenever a call comes in from an incoming patient or a postoperative patient now at home, those calls are forwarded to me; that does indeed give other nurses some release. I take such calls all day long. What do I take nitroglycerin for? Can I put a digoxin under my tongue to help the pain. I'm bleeding from my surgery. Is that serious?

Of course Mel is my life saver. Mel is my guide dog. I went to California and lived with him, taking training from 4:30 A.M. until 10:00 P.M. for four weeks. He is so much more to me than just a friend. He will gladly give his life for me. He has almost lost it twice because he will step in front of a car or do anything to save me. It is impossible to describe the strong bond that exists between us . . . almost stronger than that of a man and wife.

You were a practicing nurse. You were in ER.

When I was in ER I was a student nurse and a graduate nurse. I lost my sight before I had ever worked as a registered nurse. I have a lot of friends down there in ER. It was very difficult for me to leave that part of my life behind. Even when I had made the decision still to be a nurse—even after I took this job—I had a lot of emotional conflict. For a long time I had a real passion for ER and trauma. I felt that saving lives, starting IVs, resuscitating hearts, was the only value I had to people. But in this job I've found that the gift of love, kindness and understanding can also be of great value. I can save lives in other ways than the ER route.

It must have been horrible to find yourself going blind. Was it instantaneous?

No, it wasn't overnight. But within ten months I went from 20/20 vision to being totally blind. I had only about three months to realize the end of sight was near—the first seven months or so all my energy went into the belief that this next surgery would work. I well remember going into a screaming rampage when one doctor said "There's nothing I can do for you." I was furious that he was giving up when I wasn't ready to give up. I was totally put out that he wouldn't try to help me.

Yes, I was in my low twenties when all of this happened and I'm still in my twenties, so it has been a dramatic change.

We were in Europe, my husband with the Air Force and we had been married just one month when my vision problems began.

Boy, that certainly shows what sex will do for you.

(Much hilarity. Interviewer and nurse broke up.)

Yes, we've joked a lot about that. Everyone notices that timing and enjoys a joke about it.

Yes, it all started in Europe. My diabetes was causing a lot of trouble. We got a Humanitarian Move as it's called back to the states and spent a year in San Antonio, still in the service. As my health became worse and I had my kidney transplant, my husband wanted out of the service and I wanted to come home to Minneapolis and to the Society for the Blind here, so we took that big step.

I'm thinking of the benefit to other patients because of the terrible experiences you've had. Once again, I see what a great contribution you are making.

I hope so. I tell patients constantly I know what it's like to be in the bed. I've been on the other side of the fence more than I've been on this side. When I can tell them I've been right where they are it can be very meaningful.

I like to laugh and I put humor into my group sessions as much as possible. We have these groups of eight to fourteen people. It was a brainchild of mine and with two other nurses developed a support group. All the patients in that group have cardiomyopathy. They never get better and they know that.

At the end of our spring support session some of the people said they couldn't go through the summer without meeting again. So we had monthly meetings. These group sessions have been great.

Isn't it awkward in heart groups to have to say "Old George can't make it today because he passed away last week"?

Sometimes if it's a caring group it's good to talk about death. Everybody is in the same boat. Death is taboo in America and we don't want to talk about it. Even though some feel they are living on borrowed time, I make the point that these people have an advantage over John Q. Public who feels his life will go on forever.

It's important to me to know that I'm still helping to save lives, maybe keeping people from drowning in their own—whatever. I don't want people to think that all of my work is psychological, spiritual, emotional work. I take a lot of calls from people who need good sound nursing counsel.

I just took a call this morning from a woman who said "My visiting dad is having lunch with me now; he's taken two nitroglycerin; he's getting sweaty and his coloring is bad—what shall I do?" I am not going to say "Call the ambulance" like that. I do say something like this "It does sound as if he should be seen. Why don't you pick up the telephone, call 911 and they will help you judge whether he should be brought to the hospital. Don't you drive him by yourself." They brought him in here—he's down in ER right now. This just happened a couple of hours ago.

Sometimes I wish I were ten people. There is always so much need and all the nurses I know are trying very hard to make life easier for their patients. The days are just too short.

Shelli Nicoson, RN
Minneapolis, MN

JACK AND BILL

Jack Buckhout, a local teacher, participated in our cardiac rehab program after having sustained a myocardial infarction. His musical hobby, playing the trumpet in a band, temporarily was placed on hold during his recovery. After diligently implementing guidelines to facilitate his recovery he yearned to return to playing his trumpet. His doctor discouraged his eagerness, but Jack couldn't understand why, because he felt so good. I decided there wasn't any reason why we couldn't check this out and reassure Jack one way or the other. For the first time in the history of our program I invited a participant to bring his musical instrument to rehab. I would monitor his heart rhythm, heart rate and blood pressure while he played. We always prided ourselves on individualizing a participant's care in cardiac rehab and I felt this was another one of those opportunities that we could not afford to pass up.

Jack played his trumpet and I documented his responses on monitors. When we finished I reviewed the EKG rhythm strips and findings with Jack. Using the target heart rate parameters he used for exercise during recovery, the writing clearly was on the wall. He could not argue with the facts. It was evident to him that, although he felt well, there was every indication that his cardio-pulmonary systems were not ready to handle the demands placed upon them by trumpet playing. His original plans to rejoin his musical group for part of an evening were postponed while he continued working hard at developing a higher level of conditioning. A few weeks later we repeated the scenario. This time all systems were go. He was elated and couldn't say thank you enough. He felt encouraged and confident that first night back playing his trumpet with the boys in the band. The information was conveyed to this physician. As a result of sharing this incident with my colleagues, I later was nominated for the educator of the year award at the hospital and won! What a delight for all concerned.

While we're talking, I'd like to tell you about Bill, a male participant in his forties who became re-involved in cardiac rehab after underoing coronary artery bypass surgery for a second time in eight years. Before a very rocky post-op recovery, Bill almost died twice. Divorced, without insurance, and without any family nearby, he didn't see any possible way he would be able to participate in our program. I felt it essential that he do so and went to bat for him. I contacted appropriate people and he was granted a limited number of visits to attend cardiac rehab. We worked with him closely, reinforcing risk factors, encouraging him and offering support. He is alive today several years later, has kept off 35 pounds and is back at work paying off a tremendous amount of medical bills as a result of that hospitalization. What a happy ending.

Cardiac rehab was truly like one big family. The support and comradeship were mainstays in helping the participants maintain some hope. Our staff and participants held Christmas parties, Valentine Day dances and an annual picnic in addition to Go Big Red Days, were we held pep rallies before the first college game of the season. We had Halloween parties and participants and staff would come dressed in costumes to exercise. We loved it and they loved it. We laughed, they laughed. Photos preserve great memories and we took a lot of them. One day we had everyone wear his wildest and craziest shorts. The fun never stopped.

Current participants and program graduates from years past continue to keep in touch. The staff and participants never forget each other. Reunions are always sweet and many times reminiscences bring tears to our eyes. The participants always tell us they could never have made it without us. I feel to this day that cardiac rehabilitation is a vital link to their recovery physically as well as emotionally.

My work in cardiac rehabilitation was very rewarding and challenging. I miss it a lot. It's similar to feeling homesick but one moves on and becomes involved in other areas, seeks other rewards, touches other lives, and reaps other blessings. I'm very pleased to have had these experiences, and very grateful.

Cec Sercl, BS, RN
Lincoln, Nebraska

THE LITTLE FARMER

Fall was working its magic on southern Minnesota the day I met Johnny. Turning brilliant shades of red and yellow, the leaves were hanging on for dear life, fighting their inevitable fate, just as Johnny was doing.

I had cared for many children in my four years as a registered nurse in the busy cardiac surgical ICU section of the hospital. Patients arrived hoping for a chance to grow into adulthood . . . to share equally with others. Both miracles and tragedies became staples of my job, yet few patients would affect me as much as did this little golden-haired farm boy from Iowa. His lips may have been blue but his smile was pure gold and could melt the coldest heart.

Johnny and his parents had left their family farm in search of a cure for his congenital heart defect. He was searching for the energy to keep up with his brother and to play on the miniature tractor which symbolized his desire to be a farmer, just like his dad.

His hospitalization was complicated but he was a fighter. Without his fierce spunk our nurses would have been unable to perform many of the duties, the treatments they had to do for him routinely. Drawing blood, starting another intravenous line, suctioning his tracheostomy tube just one more time. Even as he lay there, unable to talk because of the tubes, he continued to show a courage most of us couldn't begin to equal.

NURSE

My job was to be a friend as well as a nurse to both Johnny and his parents. His medical needs were met as a matter of training but meeting his emotional needs became the real challenge. He needed someone to bring him a cherry Popsicle when allowed, or to put wheels on his ventilator and give him rides around the hospital. His view of the world was like that of a fish in a bowl.

I brought him photos of my two cats to hang on his bedrail. Stories of Winter's and Smokey's daily antics would bring a smile to his face and a bit of life into his small world. We devised games to encourage him to eat when we knew he didn't have the strength to lift a fork.

The parents needed equal amounts of encouragement and support. Their world was being torn apart—their small son fighting for his life while their lives were put on hold. They had a stoic relationship with anger naturally surfacing frequently as the weeks went on. Yet the emotions of pain and fear remained just below the surface. On rare occasions when their feelings could no longer be concealed, I listened to their fears and held them as they cried.

We shared the successes as well as the setbacks. I realized they felt they could count on me to answer their questions and to fight for Johnny's cause—if not life, then death with dignity.

The day eventually came when there was nothing else to be done. For the moment the victories, however small, had overcome the failures. He was able to breathe without the aid of a ventilator and even though his activity tolerance was low and his lips still blue, there was no longer any need for hospitalization. We trained his frightened parents in the skills they would need to care for him at home; it was the start of the necessary process of cutting the ties that held us together.

The unit held a birthday party for him before he left. It was difficult because we knew he wouldn't live to see his next birthday; it was impossible to fight back the tears that we knew he wouldn't understand. As sad as was the day, I was glad to see him freed from the world of needles, catheters, doctors and nurses. It was his chance to experience some degree of normalcy, however short-lived.

The day before Johnny and his mother left town, they came to my home to meet Winter and Smokey, two faces which had kept him smiling on those long days and nights. The cats crawled all over him as he fed them cat treats and kisses. The infectious laughter was enough reward for those months of sterile environment which had kept the poor boy prisoner.

He was home just a little over a week when his tired heart failed. He was rushed to a nearby hospital by helicopter but he didn't have any fight left. He had used it all up. I was out of town when he died but the message was waiting when I returned. His mother and I grieved together and spoke often of him. He was buried at home, the headstone etched with a tractor and the name of the little farmer who never got the chance to be "just like my dad."

He was the last patient I ever cared for as an ICU nurse. I returned to school to become a certified registered nurse anesthetist, my days thereafter being filled with nursing in a different setting.

As I look back I consider the degree of emotional commitment required of me during my years as an ICU nurse, yet I am quick to remember the satisfaction obtained. Many people discourage that level of involvement because of the toll it takes on the nurse. Yet every time I put a child to sleep for cardiac surgery I pray that when they wake up there will be someone there with a warm smile and a soft touch like what I was able to share with Johnny and his family.

Louise E. Randall, RN
Rochester, MN

BE RESPONSIBLE FOR YOURSELF

I'm a nurse at a free clinic for sexually transmitted diseases. Our main duties are in testing and counseling for AIDS antibodies. If results are positive we refer them to their private doctor, if they have one. We also have a list of doctors whom we know are treating people with AIDS. Sometimes people don't want to go to their own doctor; they may simply not want their regular doctor to know of their problem. Of course that suspicion is usually not justified. Because it can be very disappointing to have someone violate your confidence, we bend over backwards to protect the individual.

We have a heavy patient load here at the clinic. Every day we see 40 or more patients. One day last week we had nearly 100 patients

—that's like a big city emergency room. We have no control over who comes in.

Of course there is no charge to the patient. If they wish, they can make a donation but we are really a public-sponsored free clinic. People say they like to see that because it is people helping people.

Our patients vary in type and ethnic background. We have some homeless people, some everyday people, some white-collared people. There is no age group in particular either. The majority of our clients are between 18 and 40—yes even a few younger than that. Our youngest was 12 years old.

Yesterday I had a boy in the clinic who was 14—the age of my son. Yes, that is rough. It's really hard. I've gone through this once already with a daughter who is now 23. When she was 15 or 16 in high school I was seeing kids her age. I had a picture of her on my desk and these kids would say "Hey, I know her. I went to school with her." So now I'm beginning to have that experience with younger children.

I wouldn't say that AIDS is levelling off because I don't really know. There were estimates of the number of cases we would have by today (late 1990) but I don't remember those exact estimaes. Besides, that is the problem with making such projections; someone needs to keep them available to compare with actual results when the time comes.

I don't think we made that mark, though. A lot of things are causative factors for not reaching that projected level.

Record keeping is part of the problem. Look at all the people recorded as having died from heart attacks, simply because at the last the heart gave out, sometimes resulting from another cause.

Recently we started issuing to prostitutes buttons that say "I practice safe sex." We encourage them to wear them as an indication that they want to help in the fight against AIDS and other sexually transmitted diseases.

The prostitutes don't seem to resist wearing them. Probably our worst situation is when we talk to them in jails where people don't want us to distribute the buttons. It always gets a little chuckle from everyone involved.

Sometimes we give these buttons to men. When they are identified as male prostitutes, we issue them. I really don't know if they use them or not. We can't walk the streets to see if they've taken them off. I do know that a number of our nurses wear them on their lab coats at work . . . and people will stop them to ask "What do you mean by practicing safe sex?" There are about eight of us RNs in the clinic.

I also go to correctional institutions for women. What I hear there is that simple possession of a certain number of condoms in their pocket or purse is sufficient cause for arrest for prostitution. I don't know how true that is but I've heard it frequently.

I believe younger people are probably being more conservative now—turning the trend a little bit. I don't know whether that is truly a sign of the times or whether I am just seeing a select few people.

I frequently hear the statement that says when you engage in sex with someone, you are doing so with every person that person ever had sex with. That's a very effective deterrent for a lot of people. However, the young people (less than 20) are not that affected by it. They seem to be taking the same attitude as about smoking—that "nothing will happen to me."

I always wanted to be a nurse. I don't know what made me decide that's what I wanted to do, but all the way through my school years no one could talk me out of it. As soon as possible I took my training. Before taking this job, I worked in a big multi-bed hospital, where I had to pay my dues. It wasn't easy.

Probably the hardest thing I ever had to deal with was when I was first out of school. I was assigned a male patient whose wife was very close to him; she was there every day, all day long. She watched me for several days, on different shifts, doing all the things a nurse does, like administering drugs.

One day she finally asked me "How do you like being (I'm having trouble remembering the exact word) in housekeeping?" She wouldn't or couldn't acknowledge that I, a black woman, might be a nurse. I simply said "I'm not in housekeeping." So she looked at me and said "Oh, then you must be a nursing assistant?" I said "No, I'm not" and let it go right there. I wanted to speak up but didn't want to rise to the occasion. She finally said "Oh, you're a registered nurse?" to which I agreed. For a long time it was hard for me to go back into that patient's room because I was so angry with her. She had watched me do things that only nurses do. Surely she knew that housekeeping does not pass out medication and care for a patient in the many personal ways I had cared for her husband. It should have been simple for her to see that I was a nurse.

That is one of the experiencs that burned itself into my memory and which I just don't forget.

I hate it when people criticize nurses for those rare occasions when a patient wants a nurse and no one responds to the call button. I have been both a nurse and a patient; I know how frustrating it can be when no one comes around, but there are situations that the patient doesn't always know about. The problem sometimes is that the patient is apt to be overemphasizing his/her problem and is worried. Still, we nurses try to get there as quickly as possible and to assuage worries and concern.

The one thing I'd like to be sure to say about my work as a nurse—all my years as being a nurse—is that you've got to take care of yourself. You've got to be responsible for yourself. That's really true in anything you do. You hear people blaming their problems on someone else. She did this. He did that. She horsed around and now I have this problem. If people would just take control of their body and care for it—it can last much longer. Of course it can be repaired but it needs good attention and the only one who can really do that is the person himself. Don't wear it out. Treat it with respect. Use commmon sense.

I think the main thing I do is helping people—maybe not just in relation to sexually transmitted diseases—because I may move into another field some time, but it's helping people that is important to me, to teach them how to take care of themselves. That is the bottom line. I talk to young people at schools, children about 12, but any age as requested, and always try to teach that one thought—respect your body.

I have learned over the years that even when things are really tough, just be thankful for where I am and what I have. I see so many people with so many problems with which they can't deal. I only want to help them.

Sandra Graham, RN

Editor: Sandra is an employee of a community health department in a large midwestern city.

SHE INFLUENCED MY NURSING CAREER

My patient was a middle-aged woman who was chronically ill, resulting in a continued deterioration of her health over four years. Thinking back, it's not her extreme illness I remember, but the strong personality of that lovely lady.

After she died I needed to write the family a letter. I wrote it partly for myself and partly to let the family know how much I had learned from this beautiful person. I wrote it because I needed to say goodbye and this was the only way I knew how to do it.

I wrote it because she influenced my nursing career, my attitudes about life and death. I wrote it so I could have a copy to reread when life created obstacles and I wrote it in hopes of sharing . . . sharing that powerful emotion of caring, that caring which plays an integral part of nursing and is the reason I love my profession.

This is the letter:

"Dear Joe and Family:

I am writing this letter because there are certain memories I want you and your family to smile about and to be proud of . . .

As Susan's primary nurse, I was in an ideal position to witness family dynamics, which I must confess was a truly remarkable learning experience. I smile every time I hear Susan say "Joe, would you be nice!" knowing perfectly well she enjoyed a chuckle with your special sense of humor.

I also remember the times when Susan and I had heart to heart discussion about her illness—and never have I witnessed such optimism. She overcame the feelings of depression and fear and was the first person I have seen peacefully accept that her life would end. I strongly believe she was able to do this because of her deep religious beliefs and your supportive family.

You all pulled together at a very important time and made the true meaning of "family" come alive.

As you've told me, Joe, Susan made the family communicate. What a wonderful gift she left.

I will not forget Susan because she taught me and all those involved in her care about optimism, acceptance, and life. Yes, in fact she taught me more about living than I could ever imagine.

My thoughts are with you all and during difficult moments remember Susan's beautiful smile and desire to bring love to all those around her . . . and that too should make you smile.

Sincerely, Tammy."

Tammy A. Barkyoumb, RN
Waltham, Massachusetts

WHATEVER HAPPENED TO BABY JODI?

I remember when Jodi first worked in the ER, as an aide. She was working toward her RN degree but it was a piece down the road.

She was a sight to behold. She had compassion. I was struck by the depth of her feeling for patients and families. Constantly, frequently I saw her ease the worry, alleviate the concern, just by her interest in people. The soothing word, the careful hand on the shoulder, the obvious love and respect. She had it. So much so that I made special mention of it one day, saying "Jodi, you really have a way with people. You will be a great nurse." Of course she thanked me and was pleased.

She obtained her RN degree and worked elsewhere in the hospital, as a float, until the time came when there was an opening on the ER staff. She apparently jumped at the chance to return to her first love.

Those of us who work in ER feel we are a special breed, which is probably true of nurses in other services as well. But we know we are subjected to a tremendous amount of pressure and tension. Patients are not at their best and frequently can be very rude to us. Lives are at stake and nurses, as well as doctors, are fighting just to keep someone alive. When the patient has to wait assignment to an examining room he sometimes blames us, maybe even bawling us out for being slow, when we have been working at top speed.

Everybody can't take that pressure. When we have a screaming kid who really isn't in pain but perhaps scared, when we have an elderly person who may be chanting repeatedly some phrase she doesn't even know she is saying, we get tense just as do patients, because we can't stop the irritation.

So we can all see ourselves change and worry that the tension is getting to us more than we can see.

Today Jodi was triage nurse and I saw her at first hand, working under the great pressure of a very busy day.

For my money, she blew it.

When an inpatient called from his hospital room and explained that his Blue Cross/Blue Shield card had not been returned while he was in ER awaiting being admitted to the hospital, I took the call and said I'd try to locate the card. Jodi heard the conversation and barked "We haven't got time to go looking for his card. He must have given it to the registrars who *always* return it. Even if they had it, they would have turned it in. Don't waste our time looking for it."

But I did look for it, couldn't find it, so reported to the patient, who was grateful for the effort. He concluded that probably his wife had the card in her purse.

I saw Jodi keep a young girl from being processed longer than I thought was fair. As triage nurse that is her job but the child had an abrasion and was very scared. I know that she was passed up from the normal sequence and wondered if Jodi were prejudiced. The child was black. Of course I can't prove that I was assessing the situation correctly.

There were other incidents. Jodi was curt repeatedly. She was upset and unable to cope with the demands of her job—and, frankly, she needed a bath.

Now this is not the typical nurse as I know us. Was Jodi having an "off day" because of personal problems? Has her family caused her concern? Has her increase in weight caused the problem—or is it the problem itself?

No, her problems run deeper than that.

I truly hate to see such changes in a person. The bloom is off the sage and Jodi is no longer the loving person she was.

She's lost her compassion.

RN
Name withheld by request
Kansas City, Missouri

MARGIE FLIPPED HER WIG

My wife was a nurse for nineteen years at a big hospital. She likes to tell the story of when a gentleman returned to her nursing station after having a body cast removed. He had worn this cast for a couple of months and all he could talk about was having a shower again.

His nurse took him to the shower area and stood outside the shower curtain, waiting for him to finish. Finally, after ten or fifteen minutes and with the room filling with steam, he stated "Margie, I feel like fainting." His nurse pulled the emergency call switch and shut off the water. She reached for his crutches with one hand and held him up against the wall with the other arm to keep him from falling.

At this very moment a nurse was taking a group of people on tour and was in the shower area. She answered the emergency call and opened the door. There she saw steam pouring out the door and there stood the nude patient being held against the wall with the nurse's wig hanging on his crutch. He shrugged his shoulders and said "Margie flipped her wig for me."

Harlen Fiek
Rochester, Minnesota

MODERN NURSES ARE MORE THAN PILLOW PLUMPERS

While I was a senior nursing student at Syracuse University in New York, I was diagnosed as having a rare tumor following a routine chest X-ray. I was given only a five percent chance to survive.

By the time I went into the operating room, I had gone through the denial, the anger and the bargaining, and I reached a point where I said to myself "Sonja, if that's the way it is, then that's the way it is."

Following eight hours of surgery, complicated by massive hemorrhage, I was put on a respirator in ICU (intensive care unit). My nursing professors, determined that I would make it, specialized me around the clock.

The tumor turned out not to be malignant, but it had rapidly expanded in the chest and would have eventually constricted blood flow to the heart. Doctors told me that if the tumor had not been discovered, I would have dropped dead within six months—about the time I was expected to graduate.

That was some year. Transition is something I've become familiar with. Out of the 67 classmates who started out in my nursing class, only 22 of us graduated. Out of that 22 three of us were struck with fatal illnesses. One died of leukemia, another ended up in a vegetative state from a brain tumor, and I was diagnosed as having a dermoid cyst with embryonic features.

During those long months of recovery I remember thinking, "There's a reason I'm here. I need to make my life worthwhile."

Through a nursing career that spans 25 years I have found many worthwhile niches. I have done just about every nursing job imaginable—staff nurse, public health nurse, teacher, researcher, manager, consultant, top administrator—to name several.

What keeps me excited about nursing? What is the allure of a profession which has brought me all the way from my native east coast to my previous job travelling the length and breath of the country with the Joint Commission on Accreditation of Healthcare Organzations and now, finally to Minnesota?

I have a tremendous sense of curiosity. Learning new things and taking on new challenges is exciting for me. I am also a very pragmatic individual. I like looking at the big picture and figuring out what the problems are and what solutions there are to solve the problems. I'm very interested in facilitating change and leading others through transition.

In one of my previous jobs as a nurse administrtor, I found out just how liberating changes can be once trust is established. Hired as a Vice President for Nursing, a newly formed position, my job was to upgrade the nursing stature in the hospital from that of token contributor to partner in decision making. The task took considerable political as well as managerial skill. Soon after I arrived, I discovered barriers such as anachronistic policies—or no policies at all, a nursing director who was committed to managing the way it had been twenty years ago, an "Old Boy" network that consistently excluded nursing in the decision making process, blurred lines of authority, and a nursing staff who were justifiably frustrated by the lack of leadership and support for their roles.

Equipment and retention of nurses was also a serious problem; serious enough that the hospital board of trustees, in part, formed the Vice President position and hired me to do something about it. Within six months positive changes began to take root. Nursing staff, who had previously despaired over their jobs, were now busy implementing changes through newly formed committees on everything from standards of practice to recruitment and retention. Nurse managers, no longer dead-ended by inept leadership and ineffective bureaucracy, made progress with new ideas and policies. Both retention and recruitment increased. Even the "Old Boy" network began to view nursing positions much more seriously.

Through it all, I practiced my own brand of management, known as "MBWA" — Management By Walking Around.

If I am excited about nursing, I am convinced that others will be. You cannot communicate with your staff from behind a desk or a closed door. Neither can you understand their concerns. You have to make policy come alive for the people you serve. I used to say to the nursing staff, "If you wait for the other guy to do what you want, it may not turn out the way you want."

Events in health care are changing quickly. I no longer look at five-year goals; I look at two to three-year goals. Some of the issues of the moment are such things as differentiated practice and nurse management rights. The world refuses to stand still. Change is inevitable. Growth is optimal.

A nurse has much, much more to learn before she can be considered a nurse now than in the years when I was going to nursing school. She must understand the modern technology. She must be an engineer in that sense, so she can see what's going on with it vis-a-vis the patient. There's just so much more to know.

And, at the same time, the nurse has to go on nursing, in the old-fashioned sense. I think the undervaluing of the nursing profession stems from that old conventional wisdom: that nursing was just mothering, changing dressings, following doctor's orders without thinking for herself, feeding chicken soup, plumping pillows and generally comforting. While comforting and caring are still the unique something which a good nurse gives her patients, aligning these needs with the physician's orders is more crucial than ever. And that judgment must be based upon academic knowledge of the science of healing. Judgment in the skill of assessment is the unique, singular skill of a registered nurse. An RN is the constant at the bedside. The physician is only episodic. The 24-hour vigilance of the RN calls to attention the need to assess and reassess the patient consistently in order to make appropriate judgments to move the patient from illness to wellness.

That combination, the intense human contact, because the nurse is the one with the patient hour to hour, not the doctor, coupled with academic requirements, makes the nursing profession, as it is today, one of the most rewarding professions intellectually and emotionally.

Sonja Meyerholz, RN
Executive Director
Minnesota Nurses Association

IF I'D ONLY HAD THE TIME

The family had been with old George when he died. There had been the usual crying and much depression. His wife of 51 years seemed able to take his passing easier than their children. Perhaps it was because he had been such a long time dying. And Louise had been warned repeatedly that the end was not too far away. That poor old heart just couldn't take any more of the demands life was putting on it.

The boys from the morgue came with their cart to remove George's remains as unobtrusively as possible but, to me, they weren't "remains". It was dear old George whom I'd cared for so long, a nice old gentleman who had been so appreciative of everything I could do for him.

The problem was, as I began to realize, that I probably hadn't done enough. The more I thought about it as I continued with my eight other patients, I simply wasn't able to give the attention to each patient that I wanted to give. I leaned my head against the wall of the nursing station and almost swore. "Damn it," I said to myself, "they just demand too much of me—and everybody else."

It's true. We nurses today are so overwhelmed with paper work that to some of us it seems first things don't come first anymore. Oh, sure, I know that meticulous records must be kept. The physician must be assured tha the medicine he ordered was given at the proper time, and in the proper dosage. He needs to know the vital signs at various times of the day. Plus the patient's appetite, attitude and bowel habits. All of this has to go down on the patient's record, to be kept forever and forever I suppose.

But all of that takes time.

My head nurse wants to run a closely supervised unit. Her neck is so far out it's a yard ahead of her body. She's always subject to criticism if I don't perform so she has no patience with my excuses.

Did you give Mrs. Johnson her bath? How come you left Myrtle on the commode with the door and viewing window wide open? Didn't you get the pharmacist to change that medication? Why haven't you dressed #14's wound yet? Have you reported to housekeeping that mess in #16's bathroom? And get those records updated before you leave . . . doctors will want them done by early morning.

And so it goes.

I want to be a good nurse. I studied and went through that hell in order to take care of people. I want to ease their pain, to help them recover from surgery, to be there in any way when they need me. I want my very best to be a modern Florence Nightingale—but they won't let me. With nine patients to take care of (which is probably against the law), with all these new insurance records being required, with new safety factors to learn about, with possible drug interactions that I'm supposed to be watching for—it just isn't possible to be there every time I want to be—or even every time someone thinks I should be.

There goes 17's call button again. I suppose she wants another pain pill and she's already had all I'm allowed to give her.

Oh, well . . . . oh, hell . . . . "

Kathy xxxxx, RN

Dallas, Texas

MARY HID FROM THE NEEDLE

It was in 1972 and my little daughter, Mary, had been treated so often for ear infections that our physician recommended a tonsillectomy. Such procedures were much more apt to be performed in those days than they are today.

Now Mary didn't think too much of this idea. For some reason we've never understood, she hated hospitals and everything that went with them. Most of all she hated needles.

I thought I would lessen her fear by reassuring her that I would give her the pre-operative hypo myself. This was perfectly logical and legitimate since I worked in this particular hospital in Minneapolis. The head nurse agreed that it sounded like a good procedure and would mollify Mary's fears considerably. After all, her Mom would be gentle with her.

So we settled her in bed and we went to get the hypo prepared. We didn't take long and soon were back in her room—but Mary wasn't there. What a surprise! Had she skipped and left the hospital? Was she hiding down the hall with other children? We were concerned. After all, one doesn't really misplace a patient.

Before we left the room we looked everywhere—and then we found her. She was huddled under her roommate's bed. Poor kid! She was really scared.

All turned out well but the nurse on duty gave the hypo and Mom held the patient.

Of course the surgery went well and her problems were relieved.

That little darling is now a beautiful young lady. In fact she was married just last week.

Diane Hudgins, RN
Burnsville, MN

THE DOUGHNUT

It was one of those times when human bonding was subtle yet intense. Mid-winter 1988 found me trying to conduct an informal, weekly ambulatory clinic at a local soup kitchen. The faces from week to week were often the same.

For weeks I tried to persuade one man to allow me to examine his apparently swollen, aching lower legs which impeded his already unsteady gait. Each week he would sit down at my makeshift station, exchange a few words and then be on his way. He consistently refused to allow me to inspect his legs, swollen and layered with mismatched socks.

Two weeks before my makeshift station was to cease, this man sat down as usual and then proceeded to unravel his socks downward over two badly swollen, reddened and blistered extremities. Some of the stasis ulcers were weeping while others were caked with exudate. After cleansing his ulcers and giving him some basic care instructions, I thanked him for allowing me to help him.

Without a word he reached into his many layers of clothing and pulled from one of his jackets a doughnut wrapped and tied in a plastic baggie. He opened the bag, broke off one third of the stale doughnut and extended it in his hand to me. Without hesitation I shared what seemed to be a valued possession of this man.

Had I stopped to think about the doughnut's origin or the many hands it must have crossed, I may have sacrificed the smile I received and the trust I gained from that man. It was an experience, and a lesson, I won't soon forget.

T. M. McAndrew, RN, CNA
Jermyn, Pennsylvania

LOVING CARE PULLS A PREEMIE THROUGH

Carol and her husband had a son, David, who was their first child. She happened to be early. Premature is any baby born under 37 weeks. Normal gestation is 40 and we consider normal 38 to 42. Usually anything under 37 is considered premature. I think David was about 36 weeks.

Appearance wise he was very healthy but he would have these apnea and bradycardia spells. He would only come back at times. If you work with a kid long enough you can tell when you can give him oxygen — but some kids will respond and breathe when they are ready to do so. We thought that possibly David was having seizure problems, so we did an EEG on him and he had very normal brainwaves. So we then did a cat scan on him and found that his ventricles were enlarged. At that time there was no answer as to what could be done.

But after about a month's time he improved on his apnea and bradycardia spells, so we sent David home and probably about six months later Carol returned and wanted to show us how David had become very normal. Since there had been problems, we weren't sure whether or not he would be normal. We took pictures because we were all supportive of each other. Each Christmas I got a card and we kept in touch.

Three years after David was born it was time for me to leave ICU. It was my very last shift, and at night. We had an emergency call to pick up a mother and newborn twins at another hospital to transport to ours. Since it was my last night I said I'd go on the call and sort of go out flaming. Imagine my surprise when I got there and found it was Carol, three-year old David's mother. Before we went out we had only known we were picking up newborn twins. I knew she was pregnant but didn't know she was in the other hospital.

Twins may frequently come early so that indicated nothing. I saw her husband in the hospital and he said "You know what? She's going to be damned happy it's you coming to get the girls."

So we stabilized the girls and then went in to see Carol, after her husband had gone in to tell her Kathy's here. I got this really big hug and she said "I feel really good that you're going to be taking care of them but I'm sad that I can't hold them." I said "Well, maybe we can work around that."

It's important to know that it's very meaningful for a mother to hold her newborn immediately after birth; Carol had been denied that at David's birth and now wanted to do so very badly.

She couldn't hold them because one was having a little breathing problem: we discussed it and she was happy to see them under any condition. She got to hold one of the babies for a few moments. The other was not critically ill but just needed close attention for a little longer.

She was so grateful to have the opportunity to fill her dreams. She knew she had premature babies and that there was no danger of losing the other child.

Any problem is a very painful experience, because you assume normalcy. If you've had one unhealthy baby, the next delivery can be very painful, distressing.

After having been in ICU for so long and then moving into obstetrics, I have a closer empathy with mothers in that situation.

You know, when I started nursing, the public seemed to think it was always only the doctor who cured them but increasingly today I'm hearing patients say "It really was the great nursing I received which made me well." Those are mighty pleasurable words for any nurse to hear.

Kathy Kerber, RN, MS
Minneapolis, MN

A CHRISTMAS MEMORY

I was in my first year of nurse's training in 1949 at a small hospital in northern Minnesota. I had been home only once since starting school in September and was looking forward to going home for Christmas. Then the director of nurses announced that the freshman class was to split the holidays, with half going home for Christmas and the other half doing so at New Year's. Much to my dismay, I was in the group to stay at the hospital for Christmas.

On December 24 I worked a split shift; one of my patients was a Mrs. Anderson who was in her early forties and dying of cancer. In the afternoon her husband and the oldest of several children visited her and brought a small tree from the farm. It was decorated with a paper chain and pictures cut from a catalog. Because they lived several miles away they could not return that night, particularly true since more snow was predicted.

That evening, upon returning to the quiet halls of the nurses' residence, I stopped by one of the rooms where a few students were gathered. Someone had made Christmas cookies and they asked me to join them. I was tired and just wanted to take a bath and go to bed, so made my excuses. But before I could go an announcement was made that we were to don clean uniforms and meet in the hospital to sing carols. Putting together a fresh uniform with stiffly starched collar, cuffs and apron, let alone singing, was the last thing I wanted to do on that Christmas eve.

After bathing and putting on the uniform, I looked out of my window and could see a lighted tree in a nearby house. I turned off the light and stood watching the falling snow and the tree for a long time. Feelings of isolation and loneliness were so overshelming that I wanted to cry, but couldn't. How I missed my home and family, and how I regretted coming to this place instead of a normal college where people got to go home for Christmas.

However, I was soon walking the hospital corridors with the rest of the nurses, our voices raised in the familiar carols. We paused at each open door, sang a while, and then moved on. When we came to Mrs. Anderson's room, she raised up as far as her pain would permit and smiled and waved to me. Suddenly, looking at her, I realized that these were the last carols she would hear on earth, and I wanted desperately to sing on and on for her. The desolate feelings I had possessed disappeared and I sang with a renewed spirit.

The next morning when I went in to care for her, she took my hand and thanked me for coming by to sing to her the night before. Then she asked if I had gotten any sleep, because she said she had awakened several times during the night and had heard us singing, and how beautiful it was. I told her we only sang for about thirty minutes after which I had gone to bed, because I had to work early this Christmas day. But she insisted that she hear us singing during the night, and had even heard the rustle of our uniforms as we came

by, but that it was too dark in the hall to see us. There were no ra-
dios (and of course no televisions) in the rooms at that time. I
started to tell her again that it couldn't have been us she heard but
the look of radiant happiness and peace on her face stopped me.
That peace seemed to permeate my being as well and I felt what in
later years I learned to call "the real Christmas spirit."

She died the following day, peaceful to the end. I went home for
"Christmas" at New Year's but it wasn't the same. The tree was still
up and my family gave me more gifts than normal. My mother even
prepared a special dinner. However, I felt I had already experienced
Christmas in a way that made me feel somehow wiser and older than
my years.

Now as Christmas approaches and I hear certain carols I think of
the Christmas 40 years ago. I never again experienced the feelings
of isolation and loneliness as I had then, but I have always wondered
who it was that Mrs. Anderson heard singing for her late into the
silent night.

Rosalyce M. Hoppa, RN
Rochester, MN

HOW OLD WAS SHE?

She came into our emergency room in pain, a middle-aged woman
hanging on to youth by wearing mod clothes, high heels, a trim
body but overtreated blond hair and a tired, worn face.

With her was a young man ("stud" I thought) whom I had seen
before, a dark-haired muscular Italian or Jew, truly a handsome
man. We acknowledged recognition from previous meetings.
"Yes," he mentioned, "she's back again with a sprained ankle."

"Hell," I thought. "Did he throw her down a stairwell?"

Mable registered her, obtaining all the facts—address, payment
responsibility, insurance, age, job contact, et. In a few minutes she
brought me a group of stickies (labels) to affix one to each sheet of
the records we'd have for the patient.

But Mable pulled me aside, giving me one special label. "Here,"
she whispered. "Put this one on her wristband." Before I could look
at the label, where the age was inked out manually, Mable con

tinued "She doesn't want her boy friend to see her true age—which she gave us."

So Mr. Stud didn't find out that she was 53 years old—instead of whatever she had been telling him.

RN
Name Withheld on Request
Chicago, Illinois

IF THE MOTHER DIED, THAT'S JUST THE WAY IT WAS

I worked in Belize for quite a while—just south of the Yucatan peninsula. Actually we were on Ambergris Caye, an island of Belize. Everyone enjoyed pointing out that Ambergris means whale vomit and that the island was covered in that material.

With my husband, Clay, we'd been working in Texas and went to Belize to run charters off this island. It was a beautiful place, with English being the official language, as it had been part of the British empire previously.

I soon missed my work as a nurse but had no work permit. Also there was no reciprocity there to recognize me as a nurse, so I had no official standing.

There was a local doctor's office but the doctor only came for two half-day visits each week. He not only permitted me to use his office and equipment, but encouraged me to do so. I was a volunteer in health services, you understand.

I saw a lot of pregnant women and tried to help them. In Belize women just went ahead and had their babies. There was a high infant mortality rate and it seemed that if the baby died, it died. If the mother died, it was a shame, but that's the way things are.

If we had a true emergency on the island we could call for a little plane which landed on our tiny strip. If it were to be a night-time landing, the men would bring their three-wheelers and line up along the strip with their lights on.

One of those occasions I remember was when a man had his foot amputated with a machete. I don't remember how it happened, but

I couldn't handle that very serious situation. There was no surgical clinic there and, as I've said, no physician present.

The doctor's office was financed by the Lions club. I think it was the Lions International, plus the local club.

Just before we left the island, the clinic people offered me a full-time job in the clinic for $400 a month, which was very good money for that place and time. It was a man's salary and surprising to me that they would offer it to a woman, in that machismo country.

Individual families whom I was able to help wanted to pay me. They would bring us fish, although my charter boat captain had plenty of fish, or coconuts, or they would make gifts for me. I appreciated these signs of love and concern.

There was also a physician at another location, working with the support of the Presbyterian church. He had an opening for a nurse-clinician and offered it to me. Because it was inland, Clay couldn't operate his charter business there, so I had to decline. Although I still didn't have a work permit, the church could quickly obtain work papers for me without paying the fees because it was missionary work.

After about nine months we left Belize because officials there thought we were rich norteamericanos and kept increasing the duties against our charter business. When my husband objected strenuously, they thought he was bluffing and threatened to pull his work permit. Thus we had a Mexican stand-off. When we had paid them $30,000 duties in nine months, we said enough-is-enough and returned to the states.

Pam Sikes, RN, BSN
Marathon, Florida

I'M PROBABLY THE LAST PERSON
YOU SEE BEFORE SURGERY

Here is the best kept secret of medicine.

So many people think the anesthesiologist puts them to sleep and then wakes them up. A lot of people don't understand that they are never left alone for a minute. They think that the anesthesiologist gave them a drug and then left. That is true but the anesthetist takes over after the initial putting to sleep by the anesthesiologist (MD)—and they are never left alone.

The nurse-anesthetist stays with the patient. Anesthesia sometimes causes amnesia and the patient simply forgets what has happened. Both the anesthesiologist and the CRNA (Certified Registered Nurse Anesthetist) interview the patient, give a hypo, check the chart, and take him into the surgery. Sometimes the anesthesiologist pushes the medicine and sometimes we do it. We don't have enough anesthesiologists to stay there all the time because multiple surgeries are usually being performed simultaneously. (*)

I have understood that the first anesthetists were trained at the Mayo Clinic. Most of them at first were women—I think the first ones were nuns. It was thought that men would be too interested in the surgery when they needed to pay attention to the vital signs they were monitoring. So for years it was a female dominated profession. (*)

Of course an anesthetist must be a nurse. For example, it took me seven years of training to get both my RN and anesthetist degrees. I've been an anesthetist for 15 years. I was one of eight children and was lucky to be able to get any college training. I couldn't afford to go any further.

Pay for nurses and other healthcare people has gradually been improving but most of us are single parents or two workers per fam-

---

*(Ed.: This is a particular situation of one person and may not necessarily be applied as a blanket statement. Procedures vary.)

ily because we can't afford to support a family on an RNs income. Today about one third of our nurses are single parents.

Today almost half of the CRNAs are men. Many times it seems in medicine that you are given the short stick unless you are a doctor and I think male nurses are very aware of this. For this reason they have seen the financial advantages of getting more training to become an anesthetist.

I'm the person who sits right at the patient's head during surgery. Yes, I'm there all the time, monitoring all the vital signs. I've seen some weird and some funny things. We have so many more monitoring devices today that if a situation changes just a little bit we are aware of it. Yes, there are all sorts of alarms to go off if changes occur. And, of course, things can apparently be under complete control and suddenly something can change (blood pressure, heart rate, cardiac rhythm, etc.). Years ago we didn't have these things with both audible and visible alarms. Sometimes they disturb the doctor and he'll tell me to "Turn that thing off."

As for these 12 to 14 hour procedures, we don't do any of those at our hospital; most go to a specialty team elsewhere. Limb attachments are long procedures and fascinating, but . . .

. . . probably the most interesting surgeries I ever observed (if you can use that word because I'm watching my patient's vitals so closely I can't do much looking) are bowel piece surgeries. Sometimes they remove a piece, then rejoin the ends. Sometimes they make a pouch of it. Sometimes they may take a piece of bowel and make someone a new esophagus. That's fun to watch. I remember the first time I saw that procedure, the doctor said "Now we have to be sure the peristalsis is running in the right direction." (Peristalsis is the involuntary waves within an intestine that move contents forward.) Just a little difference there could throw the whole thing off. I'd have never thought of that—that it must be running in the correct direction.

How do they adjust the sizes to fit? If the bowel section is too large, they don't just cut a slit and make it a smaller tube, they just taper it at one end to fit with the other piece to which they're joining it. Of course the body parts will shrink or expand as needed. Like people with one lung who eventually breathe as well as when they had two lungs. It seems to me that the surgeons do as little as possible so nature can do its work. I think the art of it is knowing how little you can do at times.

Yes, the patient sees me before he goes to sleep and after he wakes up, but he seldom remembers.

I've seen a lot of changes in my 15 years in surgery. When I started we occasionally used an EKG monitor. Otherwise we use a small stethoscope with an earpiece like on a hearing aid so we can just listen to the heart.

We go with trends a lot. We watch the temperature, for example. If it is increasing, we check it again soon to see if a trend is developing. Of course we're working with a one-on-one basis while a nurse on a station is working with several patients. We have an advantage.

I am proud to be an anesthetist. I feel really good about myself when I'm working. It's very satisfying.

I've often thought that it's too bad the patient can't come around later and we could talk. Sometimes they do trace me down and say thanks but that's rare of course.

Our satisfaction comes from seeing the patient through the surgery and come around comfortably afterwards. That's when we know we have done the job we're supposed to do. That's when we know we are doing a necessary job as well as is possible.

We start with a barbituate, sodium pentothal, but now we are using Diprivan, which is a new drug and it works great. Sodium pentothal lasts five to twenty minutes. Diprivan lasts only two to six minutes. We use it because it's fast and comfortable and gets the patient to sleep. Then we give them a muscle relaxant and put a little tube down their throat because an airway is necessary. At that point we use a mixture of oxygen, nitrous oxide and halogenated hydrocarbon.

People sometimes ask me if there aren't times when I feel almost in control of the patient's life, but that's saying it too strongly. We're not that powerful.

Even though everything's under control and going well you know that at any second it can change and the most frustrating thing is if you don't know why it is changing — or has changed. If you know the reason then you can do something about it. Sometimes you can get an arrhythmia or even a bradychardia (pulse rate below 50) and not know what has caused it.

If a life-threatening situation seems to be developing I'm very quick to call for physician assistance. I simply don't want to take a chance with somebody's life.

After all, life is too beautiful to waste.

Mary Redfield, CRNA
Eden Prairie, Minnesota

HER SUSPICIONS PROBABLY SAVED A LIFE

I have been a critical care nurse for 14 years. I was working as the charge nurse one evening in our 24-bed intensive care unit when a problem arose.

The patient was a middle-aged woman who had arrived in our unit late that day after having surgery for sacral cancer. She was unstable after surgery, low blood pressure, cool and diaphoretic (sweating). The resident ordered blood and intravenous fluids but her blood pressure continued to be low. Her hemoglobin was dropping despite the blood transfusions.

I called the on-call resident several times and he reassured me that she would continue to receive more blood and would stabilize. I decided at that time to call the staff surgeon at home who had performed her surgery earlier that day. I reported my findings and concerns that she was actively hemorrhaging. He requested we prepare her for an emergency catscan (this is a form of radiological examination formally known as computerized axial tomagraphy) and he would arrive shortly. The scan was done and she was taken to surgery for further surgery to control the bleeding.

The surgeon related to me later that without surgical intervention she most likely would have died that night. This incident reaffirmed my belief in active patient advocacy for these most vulnerable patients.

Katherine M. Zahasky, RN, CCRN
Rochester, Minnesota

AIR FORCE NURSE FINDS HUMOR

I retired from the Air Force Academy in 1978 after 20 years of active duty, serving in nine different Air Force Medical Facilities. I've had numerous humorous situations and would like to share just a very few.

From 1964–1966 I was stationed in Colorado Springs at a very busy A.F. outpatient clinic. I was a young captain, the chief nurse and the only military nurse assigned. Under my supervision were five civilian nurses, all more experienced than I. Two of these RNs worked solely screening incoming calls and making appointments, using five very busy incoming lines.

One day a young airman called to make an appointment for his wife in the GYN clinic. Screening the call, the nurse asked what kind of problem his wife was having to which he replied "Oh, she ain't got no problem. She just needs one of those Pap smears."

The nurse then explained to him that we had a pap smear clinic every Wednesday afternoon and that she was making an appointment for his wife at two o'clock the next Wednesday afternoon. Then she added "Tell your wife no douches two days before this appointment."

He exclaimed "What?" and she repeated the instructions very slowly, carefully enunciating: "Tell her no douches for two days before the appointment," to which the airman said in great astonishment, "She can't do dishes for two whole days?"

Let me tell you about Colorado Springs. It is a great tourist area and many people come to see the Air Force Academy, Pike's Peak, the Garden of the Gods and other highly publicized scenic spots.

Into the emergency room of that same GYN clinic one day came a lady complaining of heavy vaginal bleeding. The young physician examining here asked questions such as these:

"How long have you been in this area?"

She replied "We arrived a week ago."

"How long have you been bleeding like this?"

"Oh, it started about the same time we arrived here—as I said, about a week ago."

Then the doctor asked how old she was, to which the lady replied "I'm 46."

"Have you been through the menopause yet?" he next asked her.

Her reply was "Heavens, no. We haven't even been here long enough to go through the Garden of the Gods."

These and similar bits of humor have really helped me through some of the very difficult times of being a nurse. It's been a great experience too.

Sara E. Devlyn, Lt.Col., USAF, Ret.
Hampstead, North Carolina

REAL SWEET AND RICH COCONUT PIE

As I was using my favorite recipe to make the world's best coconut pie, I remember how I came to have that recipe.

I started my nursing career as an LPN (Licensed Practical Nurse) in a nursing home in Indiana. I met many patients that impacted on my personal life and my nursing practice in that nursing home.

One such patient was Mr. Hamblin and his wife. Mr. Hamblin arrived in the nursing home one afternoon, having been transferred from one of the local hospitals. I got my first good look at Mr. Hamblin as I assisted the ambulance driver in putting him to bed, and I found those haunting, crystal clear, blue eyes staring at me with the most bewildered look. I began talking to Mr. Hamblin but soon realized he wasn't hearing a single word I was saying. The wires on his hearing aid had become disconnected during all the moving around. I spent quite a while doing my initial assessment and trying to make him feel more secure about his new surroundings. I should also add his stroke had left him totally aphasic (loss or impairment of the power to use or comprehend words) and communication was difficult.

As I left his room I felt very smug with myself because at least the bewildered look had disappeared and a smile or two had crept across that beautiful old face. My feelings of smugness were short-lived as I ran smack into Mrs. Hamblin. She couldn't have stood more than four-and-a-half feet tall and probably weighed a hundred pounds at best, with a brick in each pocket. She made her presence known from that moment on. She informed me that the ambulance driver refused to wait for her at the hospital, and she was highly upset that she had to drive herself to the nursing home. As I stood looking at her, I thought "Boy, I'd like to see her driving . . . she probably sit on pillows." I took her to Mr. Hamblin and the minute she walked into the room, he came alive. Those crystal blue eyes became alert and, oh, so loving as he looked at her.

During the next few weeks Mrs. Hamblin drove herself to the nursing home every afternoon. When it would be time for her to leave, she would start crying and he'd become restless. I decided I needed to help this beautiful old couple so I started spending time with them. I found that they had been married when he was 17 years old and she was 14 years old. They had celebrated their 75th wedding anniversary about a month before the stroke. Their only son had died suddenly five years previously with a heart attack, so they were all alone except for grandchildren who lived in a distant state.

Mrs. Hamblin and I talked about his care . . . how he liked his food, his bath, and his shave. She showed me how to dress him, just so, with his suspenders, and how to comb his hair. It was as if by including her in his care, she felt needed and content.

Mr. Hamblin was doing wonderfully with his physical therapy, and each day she was there to give him words of encouragement. She kept telling him "As soon as you can walk, I'm taking you home." I thought to myself: "You're 89 years old and you're going to do all his care?" I soon learned that determination isn't measured by one's size, but rather by one's heart. Mrs. Hamblin would sit by his bed for hours reading poetry, novels, the Bible, and letters from the granchildren. Even though he couldn't speak, they had their own language and could communicate beautifully.

She would call every night to make sure he had been tucked in for the night and that he had fresh water by the bed. She would say "I know you're taking good care of him, but I'm so lonely; tell him good night for me."

Over the next couple of months I became very close to this wonderful, gentle old couple. As the day approached for Mr. Hamblin's discharge (he was walking in the hall with a walker by now), Mrs. Hamblin thanked me for the care and support I had given them.

She wanted to give me money for helping them, which, of course, I refused. The next day she came to the nurses' station with a basket. She said that since I wouldn't take any money, she had baked me a coconut pie. Later that evening as I had a slice of pie I thought I'd died and gone to heaven. The pie was so smooth and creamy that it was wonderful. On the following day I thanked her for the pie and asked for the recipe.

On the day of discharge Mrs. Hamblin gave me yet another pie, along with the recipe. She had entitled the recipe "Real Sweet and Rich Coconut Pie." I thought, how wonderful to remember someone by a recipe, since the title so aptly described how 'real sweet and rich' Mr. and Mrs. Hamblin really were.

I'd like to share Mrs. Hamblin's wonderful pie recipe with you . . .

Real Sweet and Rich Coconut Pie

1 cup Sugar
2 eggs
½ teaspoon salt
⅔ stick of margarine
1¾ cup sweet milk
1 teaspoon vanilla
1 cup flaked coconut
¼ cup regular flour.

Beat eggs, sugar and salt. Add margaine and flour. Beat well.

Add milk and vanilla. Fold in ½ cup coconut. Pour into unbaked 9" pie crust. Then sprinkle ½ cup coconut on top. Bake at 325 degress for 1 hour and 15 minutes or until top is nice and brown.

Sharon Teixeira, RN, CNA
Kailuaa-Kona, Hawaii

Reprinted by special permission from "Riverside Nurse," Riverside Health System, Newport News, Virginia

NURSE

BABY'S HEARTBEAT WASN'T RIGHT

We forget how much times have changed.

I was a new grad fresh out of nursing school and in my first job in a hospital in Minneapolis.

One of my first patients was an about-to-be primipara (Ed.: about to deliver her first child). She was young, about 22 years of age and an attractive young woman — but one who was very concerned over having her first baby.

I was assigned to her in OB and helped her undress and get into bed. Quickly I made the usual examination, such as patient temperature, blood pressure and discussing contractions with her. At first glance everything seemed to be in fine condition, until I applied my stethoscope to listen to the baby's heartbeat.

I didn't like what I heard. The rhythm was slower than usual and as irregular as some adult patients with arrhythmias. It had been drilled into me that in such cases I should not assume or make too many decisions myself, so I called the attending obstetrician to obtain his opinion.

Doctor Johnson, more experienced than I and more capable too, quickly said "This gal has to get to surgery, right now. We must do a C-section on her now or we'll lose that baby."

So she was quickly prepped for emergency surgery and rushed into the operating room. Thank God the hospital had stand-by staff on hand, because this was in mid-evening, so an anesthetist and OB nurse were available to step in quickly.

The baby was delivered by caesarean procedures and was a fine, healthy eight pound boy. The mother was young and strong and recovered rapidly. In fact, she was out of the hospital and homeward bound much sooner than was customary in those days.

Before she left the hospital, Doctor Johnson told her that she could thank the nurse for saving her baby's life.

So this was the first time I knew that I could make a difference.

Now nurses no longer have to depend on their ears to determine if the baby is in distress. We have fetal monitoring. What a wonderful invention! Before cardiac monitoring came into existence, peo-

131

ple of all ages died because we couldn't diagnose some fatal dis-rhythmias. Many lives are saved today by newer techniques, of which this is just one.

And nurses like me are glad to see these newer tools be available, to help us in our fight to make healing easier and to save lives.

Clarissa Rownd, RN
Fountain Hills, Arizona

IF YOU CAN'T DO ANYTHING ABOUT A PROBLEM, FORGET IT

Mable Mowery has a marked Stokes-Adams syndrome, which is a problem "characterized by slow and occasionally irregular pulse, vertigo, syncope, pseudo epileptic convulsions," etc.[1]

All of which could mean fainting and/or dizziness.

On top of that, at age 99½ she was admitted to our small Band-Aid hospital with severe congestive heart failure. After four days of intensive therapy she was slowly deteriorating. It reached the point where her physician suggested the family come to see her. After all, her blood pressure was 100/0 to 20/5.

Mable dearly loved this one minister so we called him, Reverend Little, to come see her. He came, walked into her room and said "Hello, Mable, I'm glad to see you." She opened her eyes and said "I'm so glad you came to see me."

Three days later she was so well she went home. (This story can be documented if you wish—only the names have been changed to protect people's identity.)

Mable Mowery has no wrinkles and, most amazingly of all, comes from a long line of short-lived people, average age at death being between 50 and 70 of cardiovascular disease. You thought I was go-ing to say they lived long lives, didn't you? But not so.

Her philosophy is "If you can't do anything about a problem, for-get it."

She has me stumped as to how to care for her. There are many instances I could recount when it is very difficult to help her, but she is a remarkable woman.

Virginia Bare, RN
Bucyrus, Ohio

1. Stedman's *Medical Dictionary*

MRS. CATHERINE WILSON

Mrs. Catherine Wilson was my most remarkable patient. At 93, she had never been sick a day in her life, and in spite of being thin and frail, she was still a lovely woman. Recently, however, her family said she had been ill. They said she would roll her eyes, twitch and jiggle her body, and finally drop off to sleep for a few moments. They brought her to the emergency room whrere her EKG showed a bradycardia of twelve beats per minute (no, that's no misprint, twelve). Apparently her metabolic needs were so decreased that 12 a minute kept her dynamically stable enough to live quite well. In fact, she had probably been ticking away at 12 for years.

She was brought to my unit to prepare for a pacemaker implantation. Alert, somewhat anxious, she and I discussed the impending procedure. Suddenly, her pulse rate dropped to eight—so slow I relied on both my counting and the monitor digital readout. I listened to her chest and took her blood pressure very slowly. Sure enough, eight, with a B/P of 90 over God-knows-what. She was still talking to me, and denied any complaints.

Then her pulse rate was six.

Then four.

Then asystole (cardiac standstill). And still talking.

How in God's name do you CPR a person who is still talking to you? "Mrs. Wilson, can you hear me?" I asked weakly.

"Oh, yes, dearie, but I do feel just dreadful." (Dreadful! She feels just dreadful?)

I checked the leads, the monitor and her. I listened to her chest. Thirty seconds went by. Then 60. Slowly, her voice trailed off, her eyes rolled back, she had a brief seizure, and she became unconscious. Almost by instinct, I drew my fist back and thumped her firmly on the chest.

She jerked her head up and yelled "Sooooonnnnn of a biiiiittttccchh!"

I sucked air. My pupils dilated. She chewed me out.

This happened six more times in the next hour.

A while later, after much deliberation, she, her family, and her physician decided against the pacemaker. She would just go naturally to her final reward. Other relatives were notified of her impending death and started coming out of the woodwork. They all gathered by her bed, including her priest, a wonderful Irishman with a lovely tenor voice. He began softly to sing "Amazing Grace."

Sensitive to their needs, I lowered the room lights, closed the door to outside noise, and blended into the walls next to her bed. The priest's hymn finished and drifted off to a soulful "Amen." I glanced at the monitor. Twelve, then eight, then four, then asystole. She twitched. She sighed a long breath. Several relatives whispered their last goodbyes. Gently, she drifted off to heaven.

Then, quietly, her monitor showed one single heartbeat. A perfect PQRST (one complete normal heartbeat cycle.)

Like a bolt of lightning, she shot upright in the bed and declared "What the hell is going on here?"

Two relatives and the priest fainted.

With people like Mrs. Wilson I realized the world will always need nurses.

Peggy Lindsay, RN, MA
Hesperia, CA

Reprinted with special permission from "Modern Nurse," January/February 1990.

NURSING IS A WONDERFUL PROFESSION

Being able to see the humor in exasperating situations helps nurses get through the day. One of my more memorable patients was Aubrey, an elderly gentleman with multiple problems, including periods of confusion. I was working on the 13th floor of a very busy teaching institution which also happened to be the county hospital, when I received a call from the first floor information desk. "Do you have a patient named Aubrey?" "Yes," I answered. "Well, he's down here inquiring about the next flight to Paris." I raced downstairs to get him, not overly pleased at having to leave my 12 other patients. I put Aubrey in a gerichair in the nurses' station where he proceeded to hand out passes to a swanky downtown hotel and to give everyone who passed by a raise for a job well done. After a while the ward secretary noticed it was too quiet and realized the phones hadn't rung for some time. She checked and found that Aubrey had put every line on hold. A trick, I might add, we had never anticipated.

A few days later a security officer came to our floor with 25 or 30 hospital brochures on every one of which had been written "Help! Help! They're holding me against my will on the 13th floor. Aubrey." All I could imagine was seeing hundreds of these brochures floating down from the 13th floor, looking like a ticker tape parade. Of course I did reassure the officer that we didn't bind and tie our patients but I'm not sure he really believed me.

Then there are times when it really feels good to be a nurse. I came on a night shift in a community hospital in the MICU Medical Intensive Care Unit) where I had worked for quite some time. My patient's wife was there. When she saw me she said "I'm so glad you're taking care of him tonight. Now I can go home and get a good night's sleep." Naturally it's flattering to hear that trust from family.

There are also times when you know you have saved a life. A 60 year old man was admitted to the MICU with diagnosis of TIA (Ed.: transient ischemic attack—a small stroke). I went back to help the float nurse admit him because I was in charge. About thirty minutes after his arrival he sat up in his bed, lost consciousness, and crumpled. In doing so he occluded his airway and was not breathing. I quickly opened his airway and he began to breathe. Had nursing staff not been present, we might have had a full arrest instead of a syncopal (fainting) episode.

I now work as a clinical specialist in a VA hospital. Recently we had a very cantankerous gentleman who took a liking to me. He is very sick with end-stage cardiac disease and has an AICD (Ed.: automatic implantable cardio-defribillator—a special type of pacemaker). He had an episode where the AICD fired maybe twenty times. The next morning I found him in tears, which was very unlike him because he usually faced things with bravado and disdain. With the help of the ICU coordinator, we got a psychologist to see him. I visited him every day, bringing him lozenges and other little things he liked. Within a few days he was more like himself, only a little nicer. Now if staff has problems with him, they call me and usually we can get him back on track.

Claire Monzeglio, RN, MSN, CCRN
Miami, Florida

LET'S DREAM A LITTLE

It won't be too long, certainly by the year 2015, medical doctors will still be predominant in patient treatment, but there will be a new caregiver, the Nurse Physician, a position which will be recognized by the American Medical Association and the American Nurses Association. The Nurse Physicians will have a strong role in patient care and will have the authority to order treatments and tests. Physicians will be reluctant to see this position evolve but, after several years of observation and testing, it will be accepted by the medical profession.

That's not all. It is quite possible that rapid diagnostic procedures will take place in a machine about the size of a 1990 telephone booth. Complete vitals will be taken, including height, weight, respiration and temperature. Individual procedures could be obtained as ordered by any authorized Caregiver: X-rays of any portion of the body, or injections, could be ordered and administered in this comfortable diagnostic cubicle. The results will be available almost immediately, greatly hastening the diagnostic time.

Hospital buildings or health centers themselves will be greatly changed. At each entrance there will be special people movers. All a person will need to do is to take a seat in a moving chair, to press a selected button to be comfortably and quickly transported to his destination within the center. These will transport people to all areas of the hospital/center, to all treatment centers, to all visitor areas. The comfortable seats will move quickly along countersunk cables in hallways and up ramps to various floors, not unlike the San

Francisco cable car system. This rapid movement will eliminate the need for wheelchairs and will leave elevators free to be used only for transporting patients who need to be on carts or on beds.

The entire system of caregiving is on the verge of a rapidly changing, nay a shocking revolution of treatment, which can only be to the advantage of the patient.

William H. Hull, MA

VIGNETTES

The patient was hurting and, as usual, in a hurry for attention. The X-ray tech who was about to shoot him was also in a hurry. Why, I had no idea.

The tech said to the patient, a black man, "Joe, I'm going to take this fast, so if you'll come on in here, we'll take it fast."

Obviously he was rushed and talking down to the patient.

The patient was not named "Joe" and obviously resented the cavalier treatment. He quickly retorted:

"I don't care how damned fast you take it. Just take it *right!*" With considerable emphasis on the final word.

Good for the patient.

(Something from the past—source unknown)

DUTIES OF NURSES

"In addition to caring for your fifty patients, each nurse will follow these regulations:

1) Daily sweep and mop the floors of your ward, dust the patient's furniture and window sills.

2) Maintain an even temperature in your ward by bringing in a scuttle of coal for the day's business.

3) Light is important to observe the patient's condition. Therefore, each day fill kerosene lamps, clean chimneys and trim wicks. Wash the windows once a week.

4) The nurse's notes are important in aiding the physician's work.

Make your pens carefully; you may whittle nibs to your individual taste.

5) Each nurse on day duty will report every day at 7 A.M. and leave at 8 P.M., except on the Sabbath on which day you will be off from 12 noon to 2 P.M.

6) Graduate nurses in good standing with the director of nurses will be given an evening off each week for courting purposes, or two evenings a week if you go to church regularly.

7) Each nurse should lay aside from each pay day a goodly sum of her earnings for her benefits during her declining years so that she will not become a burden. For example, if you earn $30 a month you should set aside $15.

8) Any nurse who smokes, uses liquor in any form, gets her hair done at a beauty shop, or frequents dance halls will give the director of nurses good reason to suspect her worth, intentions and integrity.

9) The nurse who performs her labor and serves her patients and doctors faithfully and without fault for a period of five years will be given an increase by the hospital administration of five cents a day, providing there are no hospital debts that are outstanding.

(*Editor:* no comment.)

SATURDAY AFTERNOON

It's a busy Saturday afternoon in the emergency room. Patients are coming and going to X-Ray, the lab is busy drawing blood and ER is crowded. Two ambulances arrive at once. One contains a wreck victim and the other stretcher comes my way with a 53 year old man who has agonal respirations (Ed.: like death-agony breathing). a distended abdomen, the look of cancer, and two family members following slowly. I ask them to register him as I get him into a room (Thank goodness there's a door on it for privacy) and the ambulance attendants give me report. This man is terminal, has had a recent hospitalization for blood transfusions and the ambulance people could not hear a blood pressure. The preacher is with the family.

As I hook up his oxygen and monitor and look at his IV (infiltrated) I hope he is a no code. He looks much older than 53.

138

The family comes in. They do not want him to be coded (Ed.: meaning they are giving permission to avoid using heroic measures if death is imminent). He has had a good morning and his own preacher has visited, at which time the patient himself had said it was his time to go.

Nursing diagnosis: "Powerlessness: Perception that one's own action will not significantly affect an outcome; a perceived lack of control over a current situation or immediate happening."[1] I feel powerless, but turn my attention to the family. Do they understand what is happening?

They help me! There is a role reversal. They know he is about to die, and they stand on either side of him, holding his hands and talking quietly about the good times in his life, and how much good he did for other people. They tell me about the time he had to rent a white tuxedo for his daughter's wedding and the trouble he had fitting into it. They laugh a little, remembering. The preacher talks with them, supporting them. I'm in the corner, not really a part of all this, writing on the chart, and yet so much a part. I tell them that first his breathing will stop, and then his heartbeat—and that it probably will not be long.

Nursing goal: The patient will have a dignified and peaceful death while in the ER.

As I collect monitor strips and tape them to this record, restart his IV, listen to his chest and try to find a BP with the Doppler, I am determined that the best I can do for him is to be here, near and yet not in the way, doing only what I have to do to keep him comfortable, and yet I'm not sure I can do much for anyone. I'm powerless.

Within 40 minutes his QRS has widened, (Ed.: A lengthening of a certain part of the heartbeat as shown on the electrocardiogram), his heart rate has dropped and I summon the doctor to look at him. The family is calm and quiet. I make sure there are boxes of tissue around, just in case.

As I watch and monitor, the family tells me how good the nurses have been to him, and how little we get paid for all we do for people. I tell them that we get paid in many ways besides money. They say they know how hard we work and what long hours we have, and we are such special people because of it. How can they be so kind to a stranger at a time like this? I'm so moved. As his heart slows and I turn to tell them it won't be long now, I'm the one looking for the tissues.

His heart stops. The preacher gathers us around and prays. We all hug each other, with tears in our eyes. They leave to spread the word to the rest of the family. They leave to take their grief and joy home to grieve and to celebrate in private.

I'm a mess. I'm crying as if this were my father. I say my goodbyes as I disconnect the IV, remove the monitor tabs and the oxygen tubing. The doctor has pronounced him, the funeral home is on the way and I ready him for burial.

Goal met.

Nancy S. Maschler, RN
Greer, South Carolina

1. Kim, Mi Ja, and McLane, Audrey, M., *Pocket Guide to Nursing Diagnoses*, Third Edition, The C. V. Mosby Co., 1989.

A MEMORABLE MOMENT

I have cared for many patients in my nursing career. One gentleman stands out in my mind vividly.

Mr. K. had progressing head and neck cancer. The portion of his face below his maxilla (jaw) had been removed, a laryngectomy performed (excision of the larynx) and a dobhoff tube inserted (Ed.· a thin feeding tube). Attempts were made to camouflage this, to no avail.

He was on tube feedings. Every evening after his seven o'clock feeding we had an appointment to walk the hall. He would wear his black robe with the colorful dragon and we would stroll along at a slow pace. As his disease progressed he became weaker and two chairs were placed at the midpoint of our walk. It was here we rested and shared my most memorable moments as a nurse. Through writing, pictures, and eye contact, Mr. K. was able to communicate, able to share his hopes and fears. Here he showed me pictures of his boat and fishing trips, pictures of his wife and family and, as the weeks progressed, a picture of a handsome man, himself before the cancer. These photos were an intimate and personal part of this patient, ones he had not felt comfortable showing to anyone else.

Another evening, after we had reached the chairs, Mr. K. pulled out his note pad and, with tears in his eyes, wrote "Thank you for being such a caring nurse." This brought tears to my eyes also. We sat there in silence knowing that each of us had brought a piece of ourselves to this patient-nurse relationship.

Mr. K. has since died. I will always remember him although six years have now passed. It is individuals like him that make nursing worthwhile.

Beth Hogan-Quigley, RN, MSN, CRNP
Philadelphia, PA

THE LORD'S WORK

Recently I've had relatives of two patients come up to me and say "You nurses are the ones who pull us through" or "You should be paid more than doctors because you do all the hard work for us." Of course that is stretching it but it is good to hear anyway.

One very significant experience which I had on our intensive rehabilitation unit caused me to never again think of the most menial task we do in nursing as being insignificant.

I was kneeling down putting on a lady patient's shoes while she was sitting in a wheelchair ready to go to physical therapy. I looked up to see tears streaming down her face.

Startled a bit, I questioned her for the reason for this emotional expression and she simply said "You remind me of Jesus."

I thought "Wow! If I can get someone in touch with Christ's compassion and His care by such a simple, mundane act, I should never again think of bath, bedmaking, bedpans and, yes—putting on someone's shoes—as being boring, or something which should be delegated to a lesser trained person. Then I began to believe that nursing is the profession that is closest to Christ's heart. When he was here on earth He cared for people, touched people and washed their feet.

Then I also remember Frank, a middle-aged business executive who was admitted after having had a stroke. He was very depressed.

He had a teenager at home, a lovely wife. Now here he was coping with a left-sided weakness and wondering if he would be able to go back to work. He was young for this type of affliction and it wasn't difficult to recognize his depression.

As I placed the washbasin on his bedside table, I said "I'll bet you really feel depressed over this disability you have now." "You said it," he replied.

I responded with "That's normal — to feel depressed at times like this."

"It is?" His face brightened somewhat as I told him about strokes and how they affect one emotionally. Soon he was saying "This has really helped me a lot. Thanks very much."

A few weeks after he had gone home I saw him working out in the physical therapy department. As I entered the room, his face brightened and he said to his therapist —

"There's the nurse who really helped me one day, in rehab, when I was feeling really down and depressed."

At that time he had regained almost all of his previous functioning.

On another occasion I was feeding an elderly lady who had just been admitted to our unit. She, too, was recovering from a stroke and hadn't said a word to anyone. We assumed her speech had been affected.

I was feeding her and she was eating very slowly. Thus I had time to think between giving her bites of food.

The chaplain had left a leaflet on the table with a short Psalm in it so I asked her if she'd like me to read it to her.

She looked me straight in the eye.

"Yes," she said. Her first word to any of us.

After I read the Psalm she looked straight at me and asked "What's your name? Where do you live?"

Somehow, that simple act had put her in touch with the Almighty and the speech barrier, or maybe an underlying type of depression, was suddenly gone. She soon became more lucid and alive and in touch with her surroundings.

Many times I have found that my deep Christian faith has been a blessing.
Naomi Smith, RN, MA
Shoreview, Minnesota
Area Director
Nurses Christian Fellowship

MY MARKING STONE

I am originally from India, currently a United States citizen, living and working here for the last 14 plus years.

The year 1991, especially January 17th, inspired me to write this small marking stone of my career. (Ed.: Nurse Joe explained that she meant a reaffirmation of her desire to serve the needy all her life as long as she could.) I am frustrated from not being able to escort our troops in Saudi Arabia with my special gift and talent in two areas, specifically: 1) the ability to comfort my patient when he or she is in the desperate distressing time physically or emotionally; and 2) the ability to start an IV with 80% success rate throughout my career.

I would like to highlight one striking experience in January 1967. I was working as a nursing instructor in a government nursing school. India's adversary was dropping bombs in the heart of our city in an island which was two or three miles from the dorm of the nursing school where I was boarding. We had a general hospital close by our nursing school, the same hospital from which I was graduated. Almost all of the medical doctors and nurses knew of my special gift of starting IVs even when all the experts had failed. It was routine that I receive a call from the operating room, emergncy room, labor and delivery, even during the course of my lecture, asking me to run over and help start an IV. This is true in the USA also when I was working in a general hospital on the medical/surgical unit.

This particular incident happened in January 1967 when India was under attack. We had blackouts from 6 PM to 7 AM every day during the crisis. We were asked to sit under heavy furniture when the air raid alarms went off. On this day I was sitting under a big table, three months pregnant, and the alarm was going off. I heard a knock on my door. With no light or even noon in the sky, it was pitch black. With the high rate of anxiety from the alarm, the knock on the door really added to my fear of the unknown. Knowing of the past practice of nurses coming over to my dorm room during crisis in the hospital, I immediately ran toward the door, forgetting all about the alarm and my safety. It was the 11 to 7 supervisor's messenger wanting me to start an IV for a patient in surgery with a ruptured uterus.

I didn't care to change my nightgown so I ran three blocks, how fast I cannot explain. On arrival, to my shock, I saw a 27 year old woman with an ice cold body. She was gasping for air and with partially opened eyes, which was not comforting. The cold I felt through my body. She remains with me after all these years.

Someone handed me an IV starting kit; there was no vein either to visibility or palpation. After saying a desperate prayer to the Almighty, I took a shot. I saw blood return and all in the operating room jumped with joy.

We had no modern technique of piggy-backing solutions with a single line during those years. To make a long story short, we all worked hard together and were able to save the mother's life. This gave me the greatest comfort, especially as the mother of two myself.

The point is, no matter where we are, what the circumstances we are under, professional nurses (in great percentages) would sacrifice their lives to save someone else.

We have something to offer the world as a noble profession and nurses should take that Pride in Stride.

After 30 years in various fields (of nursing) I will dedicate my life for another 30 years if God will give me His blessing and spirit.

Nurses, march on with strength and courage. There will be great rewards ahead of you. Go on with your faith and conviction.

Tracy Joe, RNC
Toledo, Ohio

FANTASY AND REALITY COLLIDE

Mary Beth was married at the age of 14 to a man 18 years her senior, a man who wanted someone to cook and clean for him and to keep a fire in the wood stove without making a fuss. Shy and withdrawn, Mary Beth went to an environment which provided little outside stimulation. Her husband was gone during the week cutting timber in the mountains. Without television and with infrequent contact by her family, Mary Beth would turn on the radio sometimes when the silence became too much.

He never abused her physically; neither did he enrich her mind. Silent, brooding and pessimistic, he survived in a world of his own making, just as she did.

Mary Beth went to church on Sunday mornings and evenings. But shortly after entering the church her other mind took over. She could hear bits of prayers and songs but her mind would soar to other places where all was light and warmth and goodness. Her world outside kept going but the world inside her head was one of her own making. And, as the years passed, she retreated more and more into her own world, without regard to time of day or surroundings. Her family knew she was "strange" but they accepted her as she was and did little to try to reach her. Her husband just wanted his house clean, some food on the table, and was unable himself to communicate clearly with most people, never mind a shy wife.

They had a child, a little girl, who was nurtured somewhat by her father. He would come out of his shell enough to hold her and rock her in the evenings. Mary Beth's family helped a little, making sure the little girl had medical checkups and shots for school. As her daughter grew, the child becamse a parent to her mother.

So Mary Beth existed, mostly on another plane, in another world. She would venture outdoors to talk to the birds. She would hum a song of her own composition. She kept the house relatively clean except when the spiders told her not to disturb their cobwebs.

Now she is in her seventies. When our world tries to enter, she cries out in pain, lost and afraid. When her husband died three years ago, she retreated even further into her small trailer. She is able to get up and cook her breakfast and look out the windows, but is unwilling to talk to anyone. Her own mind is safe because often it is blank and she allows nothing in to hurt her. She withdraws to safety of her own making.

All was well until a new neighbor, now knowing Mary Beth, saw her crawling on the lawn talking to a blue jay. The neighbor, fearing a mental breakdown, called the ambulance to take Mary Beth to the emergency department to check her over.

Fantasy and reality collided on a cool November Tuesday when she entered our emergency department. She was moaning and tossing and turning, agitated as if in pain. We could elicit no information from her and, with no family members to help with history, we could only guess at diagnosis. Electrolyte imbalance? Head injury? Alzheimer's?

When her son-in-law arrived, we were shocked to hear him say "Ah, she's not sick. She's just putting on!" How cruel it sounded!

We kept trying to reach Mary Beth with calm, quiet gentle reassurance but she could not focus on us. She just moaned and repeated over and over, "Jesus, help me!"

A telephone call to her daughter gave us the true picture. Mary Beth had not been hurt; this was her usual mental state. After an exam by the doctor, we got her dressed to go home.

As she rolled towards the door she became lucid for a brief moment and asked "Where am I?"

Who could answer her? Was she in our world or hers?

Nancy S. Maschler, RN
Greer, South Carolina

STILL ALIVE AT NINETY

All of us have numerous stories, both successful and failed attempts, joys and frustrations . . . but we all remember dearly those patients we were directly responsible for saving. I have such a story that centers around holidays.

The patient, 85 years old, had been admitted on five separate occasions over a 21-month period.

#1. April, first year. Admitted for disrrhythmias. Treated with medications, temporary pacemaker. Diagnosed inferior wall MI (myocardial infarction) and discharged home after 14 days.

#2. Admitted nine months later for ruling out myocardial infarction.

Two days later the patient became hypotensive, developed SVT (sinus ventricular tachycardia), chest pain, disrrhythmias. This was all treated with fluids, dopamine, verapamil, lidocaine, epinephrine, Isuprel, Dobutrex, an anterior line and Swan-gang catheter was placed.

This was a day we planned a party at work (football on TV, etc.) End result was a day of constant, hard work—mentally and physically. No breaks, no lunch (the hospital provided a free meal but no time to eat), no watching television. But when we went home we were exhilarated about the work we provided. The patient was alive and we were directly responsible. The patient was discharged in ten days to another hospital for CABG (coronary artery bypass graft).

#3. Admitted two months later for syncope (temporary suspension of respiration), of bradycardia, and to rule out myocardial infarction. Later discharged with diagnosis of bradycardia secondary to digoxin toxicity.

#4. Admitted nine months later, again ruled out myocardial infarction. Medications changed and discharged within a few days.

#5. Two weeks later, admitted for R/O again. Hypertensive, chest pain, treated with fluids, dopamine, magnesium sulfate, Vesprin, Nth drip, placed Swan-gang catheter. Patient was transferred four days later to the medical/surgical floor and discharged home the next day.

The patient was hospitalized three times around the holidays; we gave him several opportunities to enjoy more holidays.

The patient remarried two years later and moved to a tropical island to enjoy the remainder of his life. He is still alive at 90.

Jerry Christy, RN, CCRN
Crescent City, California

CROSSING OVER

Death and dying have always been part of a critical care nurse's life. We live with it daily and occasionally there comes a time when we must help our patients let go and cross over.

Let me tell you about a patient I cared for, for just one day. The Colonel was admitted to ICU experiencing an acure myocardial infarction. He was a pleasant, elderly gentleman who smiled frequently in spite of his distress.

As I was admitting him, he said "I know now terribly ill I am and all I want is to see my son before I die. I need to tell him again how much I love him."

"He's been notified and is on his way," I answered. "He should be here any minute and he can see you as soon as he arrives."

Suddenly the Colonel took my hand in his. He was trembling and his color was ashen. "I'm not going to last much longer," he said as he began fibrillating. The monitor showed ventricular fibrillation . . . I believe that every patient knows when death is imminent.

I thumped his chest with no result. Then I called a code. (Ed.: Called for a Doctor Blue emergency.) The team came quickly and the Colonel responded to just one shock.

Awake now, he looked at me pleadingly and asked, "Where is my son?" I knew he needed to talk and share his fears. As the doctor and other nurses left his room he looked at me with large tears in his eyes. I took his hand and sat beside him on the bed. An overpowering warmth and gentleness flowed from this dying man.

He had been in World War II. He didn't want to fight, but felt it was his duty. The pain and agony on his face showed his deep feelings as he relived his experiences with me. As his tears began to flow, so did mine. I am a stranger to him really, just a nurse. Maybe I should encourage him to be still, to conserve his strength. He'll need it all if he is to survive until his son arrives. But he is alone now and he needs desperately to talk.

"I'm here," I tell him, "and I will listen." To myself I think "I will listen with my heart and with my soul."

He closed his eyes and began to relax, and then he told me that when the war was over he went home to his wife. They were unable to have children so they adopted a son. They named him Hal and he was to be their only child. He needs Hal now. He should be the one to listen and to hold his father's hand. But I'm the only one here, so I'll listen and try to comfort.

A nurse often knows when a patient is not going to survive, and the closeness and sharing before death is the most important part of the time that is left.

As I sat on the edge of the bed facing the cardiac monitor, I soon became aware of what was about to happen. All the skill and knowledge of a critical care nurse came into readiness and I was prepared to act at the exact second needed. I slowly got up from the bed, but he wouldn't let go of my hand. His eyes were pleading. As I administered medicine and brought the emergency cart closer to the bed, I saw the other floor nurses coming through the door. They had been watching the cardiac monitor and were ready also. This brave man now looked at me and said "I don't feel right. I'm getting dizzy. Where's Hal? Where is my son?"

At that second he again went into ventricular fibrillation.

Shock once! Shock twice!

Thank God he came back again. "Not for long, though," we think, as we all look at each other.

When the Colonel finally opened his eyes, the first thing I saw was his sheer panic. He grabbed at everything until he found my hand. And then as he looked deeply into my eyes, he squeezed my hand and said "It wasn't so bad."

It's not so bad . . . to die!

Then he explained to me what had just happened.

"I was feeling dizzy and a fog came over me. I could hear your voice above all the others. You were saying "Hold on, it's not time yet" but your voice faded. It was green . . . everything was green and I thought 'Where am I?' But then I knew I was in a forest, a beautiful gree forest, just like the one I've always wanted my son to see and walk through and breathe deeply of the fresh air. It was so peaceful and warm and the sunlight was streaming through the branches of the trees. There was a great calmness and a deep peace came over me. I started walking to the edge of the forest toward a brilliant white light. It was as though I were floating, my feet wouldn't touch the ground. I had no weight.

"As I walked to the edge of the forest thoughts of my son and my wife who died long ago flooded my mind. I kept remembering I hadn't had time to tell my son that I loved him and was proud of him. And most important I think, I knew that now I must tell him that I was no longer afraid of death.

"As I was about to the edge, I could hear your voice again. You were whispering quietly and calmly in my ear. You told me, "Hal is here. It's not time for you to go yet. Hal is here." And so I started to walk back through the forest, but my legs and feet seemed much heavier. Walking was much more difficult, but I finally came out of the fog. But now the physical pain I feel is almost overwhelming me. I know my time is now very limited, but I also know that it's OK! I'm not afraid to die."

Understanding what was happening and receiving an order from the physician, I medicated my friend, knowing he would not be with us much longer.

The Colonel was crying and trembling now . . . and so was I. In some way it seemed that pure love was radiating from him. And then his son walked in. The other nurses had updated him on his father's critical condition.

I started for the door to leave them alone together but they both asked me to stay. I cleared a spot for Hal to sit next to his father on the bed and showed him the best way to hold his father. The story of the forest and the light was repeated. And most important, the Colonel told Hal he had accepted his death and was not afraid. He did not want life support measures. To die with dignity and with peace were his last wishes.

"It's getting foggy again," he said, "Please don't let me go just yet: please bring me back. I need to finish my story and I need more time with my son." His eyes were very pleading again and I could only promise that we would. I knew that was a promise I might not be able to keep. But the Colonel knew the end was near and his will to survive a few more minutes would make the difference.

It took much longer to bring him back this time. There wouldn't be another time. I lost count of the times we shocked him. The doctors wanted to intubate him . . . to put a tube down his throat to breathe for him, but that meant he wouldn't be able to talk to his son. The anger I felt consumed me. He did not want this. It would be so unfair to both father and son.

"Lord, they know he is dying. Please let him have these precious moments with his son. This time is so important. It's the only thing that's left for them. Dear Lord, please let him wake up one more time."

He did.

We all knew that death was very imminent. His eyes were glazed and his grip much weaker. I leaned close to his ear and said "It's OK. Hal and I are here and we love you."

He opened his eyes and they cleared a bit. They had been strong blue eyes, full of power and determination, but now they were weak and full of tears. He said he was at the edge of the beautiful green forest this time, and walking into the light.

Hal looked at me and we were both crying. The Colonel's love of life had been so strong and now he was about ready to leave. He had accepted his death and was very calm now. It's a calmness that comes only when there is no longer any fear.

"As I walked toward the light I saw your mother," he said, looking at his son. "Don't cry. She's fine and beautiful as I've never seen her." And there was a faint sparkle in his eyes. "Hal," he said, "you've brought me so much joy through my years, please don't grieve for me. I'll be fine and I'll be waiting to greet you later. The white light was so soft and warm. I knew it was the Lord and a deep calmness began to grow inside me as I walked toward Him . . . a deep peacefulness . . . I'm not afraid now." Then he looked at me. "Please don't try to bring me back. I'm ready to go and be with my wife. Hal and I will miss each other, but my time is now."

We both knew the Colonel was saying his goodbyes. Hal held his graying father as a father would hold his child and quietly whispered to him, recalling all the special, wonderful moments they shared. He spoke of his fears, his triumphs and the love and joy they had known. He told his father how much he loved him and how much he would miss him. But, most important, he understood his father's last wish. To die with dignity and with peace in his heart and his son at his side.

I whispered to him, "Your son is with you and he is holding you.

Remember the forest and the meadow. We know you are in the meadow now and with your wife and your Lord. Let go of these earthly ties. Your son loves you and he is letting you go. He understands because you have taught him about life and about love. Let go . . . you've fought a good strong fight, but now it's time to let go."

As Hal and I watched the monitor, slowly . . . there were no more heart beats. He had finally crossed over. He was at peace.

And briefly, until the next time, so was I.

Laurie Vassel, RN
Charleston, West Virginia

A TALE OF TWO PATIENTS

The Charles building is a haunting edifice—the oldest section of the hospital. Patients were never happy to be admitted to these rooms. Their complaints started at the first glimpse of the dirty peeling paint chips, the antique olive green oxygen tanks and the general absence of wellness which pervaded the halls.

This tale takes place on a night shift in the Charles. Sounds of banging pipes and moaning patients interrupted the usual silence that occurs from midnight 'til dawn. On this particular night the spirits of the Charles building were very restless. At 2 A.M. a new admission arrived from the neighboring eye institute. Upon admission, opaque patches covered both of her eyes. She knew her name, denied discomfort and answered all questions lucidly. Yet when she was admitted to her private room, number 306, things began to change.

Room 306 had been occupied by Mrs. Webster who passed away on Christmas day. She was a sweet, quiet woman. Each morning, in order to help the next shift, Margaret, the LPN (Licensed Practical Nurse) on night shift, would bathe this elderly woman and lovingly brush her hair. After Mrs. Webster had been changed into a fresh hospital gown, Margaret would place a purple velvet ribbon on her head to keep the soft gray locks of hair away from her wise and aging countenance.

Once admitted to room 306, the ophthalmic patient became extremely anxious. She told us she had to get out of the room because she was not alone. Someone was in there with her. She described this person as an elderly woman with a purple bow in her hair.

Since there was absolutely no way to counsel this patient, at 6 A.M. a new room was found for her. The medical field, being what it is, also gave her a dose of Haldol. The ward clerk, quite hysterical by the incident, called the priest to exorcise the room. Today the Charles building has been completely renovated. I wonder how Mrs. Webster likes it.

Then there was Mavis who, unlike the majority of open heart patients, did not do well. Unable to wean her from the respirator and unable to maintain a viable blood pressure without the assistance of medication, we kept her in intensive care for three months. During this time I was her primary nurse.

Mavis was my personal challenge. I wanted to see her get better. Together we worked on her breathing exercises in order to coach her off the respirator. Her trach was suctioned and kept free from infection. She was out of bed in the chair every day, sometimes at the expense of my lower back. As she began enteral therapy, we both endured her bouts of diarrhea and G. I. bleeding, always trying to maintain her dignity. By the end of the three months, we had become friends. I could see her eyes light up when I approached the bedside. My thoughts were that she knew she would get good care from me.

Then the day came for Mavis to be transferred out of intensive care. As sson as this sweet woman left, another patient was admitted to her bed, another open heart, requiring a nurse's undivided attention. Memories of Mavis slipped from my mind.

One month later I was asked to fill in for a sick call on a general ward. During report I was told about a patient named Mavis. Ecstatic to see her, my night shift rounds began with Mavis. In her room I found an old woman sitting on the foot of the bed, eyes bright, breathing unlabored.

"Mavis," I said. "Do you remember me? I was your nurse when you were in intensive care."

"No, my dear," was her reply. "I was very sick when I was in intensive care."

Initially I was saddened by her response, my nursing ego bruised.

Actually, she was very lucky to have forgotten her experience in ICU. My challenge now was to help her get better, not to be her heroine.

Sherri Becker, RN, MBA
Wyndmoor, PA

THE BEST PART OF ALL

I have worked in a medical and surgical intensive care unit in a large hospital for 10 years. I was a primary nurse for a 49 year old patient who had his second coronary bypass surgery. The patient's heart was damaged from previous heart attacks. He was on and off life supports such as ventilator, intro-aortic balloon pump, and IV medications to maintain his blood pressure. He was placed on a University heart transplant list but his blood type was difficult to match and a donor was never found. The physicians were very supportive of the patient, his family, as was the nursing staff. I became very close to the patient and his family.

For obvious reasons he became very depressed and even requested his family no longer visit him. He became so withdrawn that I expressed my concern that he was not ventilating his feelings and offered some support. He replied that he thought that I was a good nurse. This meant a lot to me after caring for him for two months. The next day he called the chaplain and planned his own funeral. I attended his funeral on my 31st birthday. He was a brave and loving man and I will never forget him.

Another experience I cannot forget occurred when an 18 year old male was in a car accident and fractured his cervical vertebrae and had a closed head injury. He was comatose on arrival and over a few days gradually awoke. I was assisting him with his first meal. His orientation level was not good so it was very exciting to hear him say after his first bite, "Ish, get me some real butter." He was raised on the farm with fresh butter, so the taste of margarine was very noticeable to him. This was the first sign to his mom that her son was going to recover from those very severe injuries.

Then there was the time when a physician's car phone helped save a critical situation. The physician had pulled the post-op CAB (coronary artery bypass) patient's IV lines and had left. The patient developed a sudden onset of shortness of breath. After I assessed the patient it appeared he was experiencing pulmonary edema. I could see the physician in the parking lot and paged him immediately. He returned the page from his car phone and returned to the unit immediately. IV lines were reinserted and appropriate medications were given. The patient recovered with no further problems.

I think the most exciting experiences in critical care are the team efforts made by all health care professionals in emergency situations. Opening a bleeding post-op CAB chest in intensive care takes a team effort. This includes the on-call resident who opens the chest, finds the bleeder and sticks his finger in, as the dike in the dam story. The OR nurse who assists with equipment needed, nurses pumping IV fluid and blood and notifying the cardiovascular surgeon and the OR of the need to return to surgery. Best of all, the patient survived.

Nancy Hemmah, RN
Burnsville, Minnesota

COULD SHE FORESEE EVENTS?

I work in coronary care as well as intensive care. One day in Coronary Care we admitted a little old lady from a nursing home, admitted for a *rule out* of a heart attack. A rule out of a heart attack is a common diagnosis for admisssions to a coronary care unit. Since a physician cannot definitively diagnose a myocardial infarction until a series of blood tests confirms or denies the presence of cardiac muscle cells in the blood, one cannot diagnose a heart attack on admission. Therefore, patients are called either "rule-outs" because no heart attack has been confirmed yet, or "rule-Ins" if an attack has been confirmed by tests.

She was tiny, skinny and very spry. Also, because of her confusion, we had to tie her into her bed. According to her history, she had been confused for a number of years.

We were amazed over a three-day admission because she would request bizarre things and, for no apparent reasons, she would receive them. It was almost as if she could foresee an event or cause action. For example, she demanded to see a priest, but she was Jewish. Within minutes the staff priest walked by her room. On another occation she called out loudly for a Dr. Pepper and one appeared mysteriously on her lunch tray. Because of her struggles, her heart monitor alarm would go off suddenly and she would yell "Someone get the 'phone" . . . and then her phone would ring.

On her last day in the unit she constantly screamed "I'm going to die! I'm going to die!" This, of course, made us all nervous, particularly the plumber who was present to fix the leaky faucet in her room. As a group of nurses and doctors were standing outside her room waiting to start rounds she again screamed "I'm going to die but first I need a drink of water." Imagine the plumber's expression when a half dozen professionals burst into the room, all yelling "DON'T give her any water." No one gave her water. She did not die then and there and we were able to send her home.

My proudest moment came when I was caring for a cancer patient with a massive abdominal infection. This poor man was being given an incredible amount of blood pressure medication to keep him alive. We couldn't give him much pain medication because it lowered his blood pressure even more. He was in such incredible pain that we could read the sheer panic in his eyes. We wanted to medicate him better but that would require *levelling* him or ordering that no additional life support be given. That, of course, would require family consent. Levelling is another way of classifying a patient as a DNR (Do Not Resuscitate patient). At my institution we have five levels of intensity of care.

I talked with his wife and children, gently steering them toward realizing his true condition. After much discussion, everyone concluded that his comfort was extremely important. The long and short of it was that he and his family had a long and lovely parting, with him passing peacefully and free of pain. I knew I alone made the difference in these peoples' lives. I'm pleased to do it.

Lisa A. Kyper, RN, BS, BSN
Harrisburg, PA

MY BEST CHRISTMAS GIFT

It was several months before the Christmas holidays several years ago when Father H, an elderly priest, came to our CCU with an acute heart attack. His course of recovery had been fairly uneventful until one day, as he neared discharge, he suddenly had a potentially lethal cardiac arrhythmia. I was in charge of the unit that day and was responsible for watching the patients' cardiac monitors.

When I saw his arrhythmia I knew immediate action was necessary. I directed one person to call a code and ran to the Father's room while directing another nurse to bring the code cart.

I found Father H completely unresponsive, without pulse or respirations. He had no intravenous line up to allow any type of IV medications to be given quickly. I knew there was only one thing to do in order to save him; that was to apply paddles and shock him without delay. I did so and after one shock he regained a normal cardiac rhythm, pulse, and respirations. Appropriate care followed; he recovered and was soon sent home.

This was not the first or the last time I'd had such an experience, but something made this experience particularly special. During the following December while doing my holiday shopping at a local mall, I was walking through the mall and suddenly saw Father H walk out of a store dressed in full clerical attire and carrying an armload of wrapped Christmas packages.

I stopped right in my tracks. He didn't see me and I didn't want him to. I just wanted to savor the moment of overwhelming pride, happiness, and satisfaction. I felt I had just received a far more wonderful Christmas gift than any amount of money could ever buy.

Christine Slauenwhite, RN, BSN, CCRN
Bay Shore, New York

DON'T CALL HER "HIM"

Here are three events I can't forget.

I was caring for a hermaphrodite patient in ICU who was admitted for drug overdose. She was paranoid and uncooperative. She also looked more male than female, which explained why the staff had such difficulty calling her "Jenny," her name. Or referring to Jenny as "her." She became so angry when references were made to "him" or "his" that our staff made a concentrated effort to call Jenny "her." Since we could not use drugs to calm her, because of her drug overdose problem, we used the strategy of contagious calmness. It worked and she became more calm. She grew to trust me and by morning she was the one who initiated contacts to seek further emotional help.

Once I cared for an aged patient with a leaking cerebral aneurysm. When the patient became more sleepy about 3 A.M. the general practitioner physician said to continue monitoring the neurological status until morning but "don't bother the neurosurgeon until morning." I called the neurosurgeon and we prepped the patient for a stat cat scan, which was followed by stat surgery. The surgery was successful.

My husband, David, is a male nurse. One time he responded to a code red (fire) on a medical-surgical unit around the corner from the ICU where he was working. He was able to jump over a bed which was stuck in the door, close the window which was contributing to the fire, and remove the patient from the burning bed next to the window. After the patient was transported to the ICU where physicians cared for him, David returned to the room to assist security and the nurse to extinguish the fire. While the patient was being transported, security had opened the window to clear the smoke and the mattress had reignited.

Barbara W. Girardin, Ph.D., RN
San Diego, CA

PATIENT DISCARDED PILLS

One of my most memorable nursing experiences was with a 76 year old female patient who was a frequent visitor to our medical-surgical unit. Mrs. Q. suffered from congestive heart failure, chronic obstructive pulmonary disease and diabetes, which caused frequent ulcers. She and I had become quite close over the two years that I saw her. I knew her family members well and she knew about my then six year old daughter, Angela.

On one admission for exacerbated COPD (chronic obstructive pulmonary disease) Mrs. Q. was so short of breath that she could barely speak. Taking medications by mouth was an extremely difficult task for her. Knowing that we were always short staffed, she insisted that we leave the cupful of pills so that she could take them at her leisure. As I passed her room I would check on her progress. The process would drag on for over an hour.

One day her husband confided in me that she frequently discarded the pills after we left the room. I alerted the other shifts so a constant pill vigil could begin. Mrs. Q. was quite a story teller. She loved the extra time to tell her stories to the nurses, but felt guilty about taking up so much time.

Although standing guard did insure that the medication was taken, it made the nurses behind with their other patients.

One afternoon I was in a hurry to get out on time. She knew that I had to pick up my daughter from daycare and I liked to be there on time. I gave Mrs. Q. the 2 P.M. medications and began the waiting. She said to me, "Linda, please help me take these pills so you can finish your work on time." Knowing that she had a weak spot for children, I thought for a moment about what I could do to help her. On impulse I said "Mrs. Q., my daughter is waiting for me at daycare. If I don't arrive on time she begins to worry that I forgot to pick her up. She sees the other nurses pick up their kids on time and when I'm late she frequently is in tears." Then I smiled at her. She paused, smiled at me, picked up the cupful of medications and downed them with a big gulp of water. We were both so surprised

159

and happy we began to laugh. I gave her a big hug and then finished my shift on time.

From that day on when she had her medications in front of her, she would ask me to tell her my story about needing to pick up my daughter. We would both smile, I would tell my story and then the pills were taken with ease.

I still don't know how it happened, but two weeks after I began the storytelling to Mrs. Q. I had to take an aspirin for a pounding headache. I had never experienced any problem with medications but, for some reason, I thought of Mrs. Q. and I couldn't get that pill down. I had the pill in my mouth until it began to dissolve. I felt like I would choke if I tried to swallow. Somehow, with a big gulp of water, I finally swallowed what was left of my dissolving aspirin.

On Mrs. Q.'s next visit I asked her if she had put a spell on me. She was puzzled and asked what I meant. I told her about my pill taking experience. She laughed hysterically at the thought of me having the same problem after I had worked so hard helping her. She never forgot the incident. In fact, it became one of her favorite stories—to tell her visitors and nurses for months to come.

Linda S. Hagan, RN, BSN
Woodridge, IL

MY ATTEMPTS TO CHANGE NURSING

We all have decades when we just can't get it together.

In my twenties I was an energetic and motivated wife, mother and nurse. I wanted desperately to contribute to my happy marriage, the success and health of my kids and to my exciting nursing career. I could do it all; in fact, I think I did. All except sleep. For ten years I didn't sleep. I was so busy being the ultimate woman.

In my thirties I realized I needed more rest. I would be more willing to smell the roses, enjoy my kids more and give my husband some space. I would reward myself by continuing my education. I would draw inward and expand my worth and self esteem. I did indeed take time out. What I found was that hot house roses didn't smell as nice as the real things which were left dying in my garden while I rested. And my family did just as well on TV dinners.

By the time I was forty, I was awakening from my stupor. What I saw disturbed and surprised me. The national face of both nursing and society was changing rapidly and I found myself motivated once again to contribute. So, I looked around for something to which I could contribute.

My husband was a wise and mature business man who needed me as a wife and friend, but did not need me to view him as a cause for social change. My kids were nearly adults and preferred my contributions to be in cash only. My friends were settled and happy in their lives and preferred social rather than zealot visits. I volunteered my nursing skills for an international disaster relief agency but they never called me except during fund raisers. Radical groups were out for me. Even my dog only needed me to take him for walks on a leash which he could easily pull from my hands to chase his most hated neighborhood cat.

I guess life was pretty good for most people.

Nursing, I knew, still needed me. I saw little cracks in the infrastructure (I love that word) of my most favorite profession. Women were not being attracted as much to the big three (secretary, teacher, and nurse). They were becoming astronauts, engineers and computer whizzes. Men persistently clung to non-nursing careers, even though nursing salaries were outgaining many traditional male jobs. Older nurses were going into consulting, teaching or cushy insurance jobs, away from the bedside. Paperwork was killing off the weak.

More nurses leaving the patient, fewer coming in; this was just what I needed to get my teeth into. I could make an impact. I still had energy and time on my hands. I decided there and then to solve the nursing shortage.

I quickly planned my strategy. I would learn all the problems associated with nursing and its shortage, find out who is doing what to solve the problems already, fix everything personally—and retire.

For several years I read, studied and went to Important Meetings. The scope of the whole issue was a bit overwhelming but the hair dye was holding back the grey quite well, and I had switched to a reliable moisturizer for the wrinkles. I could solve at least some of the problems before I became ancient or senile.

The overall picture was bleak, if concise. Nationally we needed more nurses. New technologies, newly-opened doors for women and exciting never-before-developed careers were enticing teenagers and young adults away from the Big Three, particularly nursing.

In response, nursing salaries and benefits were expanding, albeit haphazardly. The supply and demand theory really was helping to shape nursing as a career. Unfortunately, it was too little, too late. Why be a nurse at $40,000 per year when you can be an environmental specialist for private industry at $60,000, with basically the same investment in education?

So, nationally we turned to sprucing up nursing as a career. State boards of nursing studied various problems and issues, and proposed various solutions. A major proposal by the states concerned itself with early recruiting and financial aid. Hit 'em in high school, or earlier, with the bennies of becoming a nurse; then provide sources of money to get the education. Likewise, for those already out of high school, such as the unemployed, the underemployed, or their parents, offer transportation, grants or loans, babysitting and encouragement.

The years it took me to get a handle on all of this was long enough. I was not getting any younger. It was time to act.

I turned to my national nursing organizations, prepared to offer help by devoting time and energy. I figured I had eight hours per week I could give these groups. I marched in, motivated and dedicated.

Aside from a podiatrist's heaven of bunions, what I found was discouraging. On a national level, we do a great deal of discussing and re-discussing, some hard lobbying and printing of much literature, not all of which is relevant to nursing.

We research and report a sea of previously studied issues, from health to politics. We educate the cream of the crop to the doctorate level, who then never again see a sick person. We publish many articles or journals written by nurses, but none written by a nurse with only an associate in science degree or two years' experience. It appears that we are only interested in the thoughts and conclusions of those who are nursing's elite.

In spite of my relative anonymity on the national front, I was eventually assigned to the job of lobbying a local politician who, it turns out, never answered my calls, never was in his office, and finally got kicked out of office. This was big league stuff for an ordinary nurse like me, and I was intimidated by it all. Besides, my time was precious, and I wasn't getting any younger. I decided to drop this national stuff and go for the state-level work.

I was still prepared, though less energetic, to devote eight hours a week to solving some of the shortage problems. Remotivated and rededicated, I marched into statewide groups to offer my help. What I found was the same bad feet, but at least things were a bit less discouraging. When I could ignore the reprints of the rehashed literature, I found at least more patient-centered activity. Many nurse-promoting, patient-caring groups existed. Some studied and promoted only specialized activities, such as critical care or neonatal nursing. Other addressed only educational or care delivery issues. Most, if not all, were genuinely promoting both patient care and the importance of nursing. Unfortunately, none communicated much to the other, and overall efforts to reduce the shortage were lost in the confusing and exciting growth of specialty groups.

Even academia is blurry on its stance. Do we raise the standards of the educational preparation to promote professionalism, or do we lower the requirements to attract more students? What results is a two-year program that takes three years to complete, and an expensive and time-consuming program to obtain a bachelor's degree. The master's degree beats a nurse to death with special projects and huge homework assignments. If a nurse manages to survive a graduate degree and goes for a Ph.D., she or he is then in an even worse spot. While being more visible or more influential, the owner of a Ph.D. earns an annual salary often lower than that of the bedside nurse.

Well, this is a hell of a pickle.

I did devote many hours to the state-level specialty groups. Within these groups I found motivated professionals, occasionally splintered by the bedside-vs.-nonbedside nurses, but always pro-patient. I found that no one seemed to be looking at what a nurse does all day, or could do if some non-nursing jobs were given to others. I also found many seminars. Seminars are excellent fund raisers and great places to network, but they do have drawbacks. Generally the same words are spoken for each topic and always—always—lunch is that horrible chicken stuffed with cheese in the middle and a pile of dead green beans. It's no wonder we get so bogged down.

This would not do. Our numbers were not increasing. Those with experience and advanced degrees took flight to better, easier jobs in management, consulting or private industry. Those with less education or experience worked even harder, then burned out.

I left the local groups. I was running out of energy and motivation. I was running out of time. I was hoping to retire in a few years.

At work I saw nurses who were running out of time too. They answered phones, they ordered and stocked supplies, they arranged for equipment, all this while patients waited for them. I saw massive amounts of paper work, frequent and mundane interruptions and high patient loads. I saw very tired nurses.

I turned finally to my last best hope. Not national, not state, not even local. I turned to the neighborhood. A darling sixteen-year old down the street was in a quandary about her future. I talked to her about nursing, both the job and the benefits. Two years later she was accepted into a fine nursing school, only to be come pregnant and drop out. Birth control was not part of Nursing 101. She wants to resume her education in a couple of years. I still talk nursing to her between diaper changes and colic advice.

A friend who is over forty and raising two kids wanted to become a nurse. We talked at length about the job itself and as she moved through her education I even tried to get her a part time job as a student nurse aide where I work. So far the job has not materialized and I'm left with the feeling that I should recruit for someplace else.

My cousin in Visalia spoke to me five years ago about nursing as a career. I sent several books to her and a job description. We talked repeatedly about wonderful patients and other nurses I've known. She graduates this summer, alongside her youngest son.

I spoke to a few groups here and there in the community about nursing. I told my favorite grocery checker about the wonderful aspects of nursing, including the ever-increasing salary. She was so impressed she dropped my eggs, which leaked down into the automated scanning device. I sold my favorite bank teller about nursing. I told my sister-in-law too.

At one point, I found myself trying to convince my husband about a mid-life career change to nursing. From that moment on, I was banned from discussing it in our home.

But, I continued to persevere. I even went on a TV talk show. The camera made me look horrible and I nearly threw up from the tension. Afterwards, I managed to polish off three hamburgers and two brownies, which eventually did make me sick.

I see no other choice for me. One-to-one, that's the only way. If I had been more awake a couple of decades ago, I would have started then. Now, time is much shorter.

If I only had the time, I'd revamp how we encourage our kids to choose and excel in a career. If I only had the time, I'd redesign our nursing educational programs which either have waiting lists or close down from lack of students, to truly accommodate a two year program. I'd change the advanced programs to accommodate the nurse who wants to remain at the bedside and maintain psychological health. I'd raise salaries to compete: I'd talk banks into loaning funds to pre-nursing students with a long payback and reasonable terms.

If I only had the time, I'd start going to elementary schools and telling the children stories about the incredible patients I've known over the years.

If I only had the time, I'd convince men how badly we need their skills, their brains and their dedication.

If I only had the time, I'd outlaw chicken with cheese in the middle, too.

Relieving the nursing shortage may indeed have to be solved one nurse at a time. I could do it—I know I could—if I only had the time.

Peggy Lindsay, RN
Hesperia, CA

PLEASE, GOD, NO EMERGENCIES TONIGHT

It was twilight in the twelve-bed ICU as I began another night's shift. The lights were dim; the monitor alarms were reset on low; in the backgrond a symphony of cardiac monitors endlessly chirped out the heartbeats of each of our patients as they rested for the night. I tied up the neck of a patient gown that I wore over my uniform, part of my nightly ritual in an effort to stay clean as well as stay warm, because our unit tended to be chilly in the pre-dawn hours. I offered a silent prayer that the shift would be a quiet one. "Please, God, no emergencies tonight." With that thought, I began my hourly tasks.

I smiled as I recalled the words of a silly tune we used to sing in nursing school, I squatted at bed #8 to drain the hourly output from my patient's Foley bag and marveled at the accuracy of our lyrics. Years of study and preparation for this! Ever so precisely I transferred the straw-colored fluid into my graduate. Slowly I rose from my chore on the floor and met a pair of eyes, round and frightened, looking back at me. My comatose patient was now awake and his eighty-year old massive black body was trembling as he tried to speak.

"Sk . . . Skuse me, Miss, but . . . is you an angel?" he whispered.

My jaw dropped a bit, and I paused an extra second to react to his question. The blue glow from the monitors, the semi-darkness, and my ridiculous gown, coupled with my patient's cardiac arrest earlier in the day, added up to one likely conclusion. This must be heaven.

Setting aside the urine, I instinctively reached around the huge chest to hug his very alive self and to carefully explain the events of the day. He listened to every word and seemed to understand, with a nod and a weak smile that this was a hospital and I was his nurse, not an angel at all.

I asked if there were someone I should call to share that he was awake. Were family members waiting for an update? "No, no missy . . . no one to call. No family, no one waiting." And he drifted off to sleep.

Each hour as I approached his bedside, he awoke briefly and would share a sentence about his lifetime, a decade at a time. It was as if he prepared a message for me each hour as I tended the other patients and, episode by episode, I learned the highlights of his existence.

As usual, the last hour of our shift had a quicker pace as we scrambled to prepare for a busy day in the ICU. My new friend slept through his last set of checks. I tried not to disturb him, but wondered what his next message might be. I gave his large black hand a gentle squeeze and reported off for the night.

I returned to work for the last night of my stretch. A shift off was long overdue. Wearily, I listened to report with half an ear, as nothing much had changed from the night before. The evening nurse included a message that the gentleman in bed #8 had expired at 0800 . . . and went on with her report.

From the nurses' station I looked out over the orderly ICU. My eyes lingered over the very vacant bed #8 as I slowly and deliberately tied up my cover gown. I took a deep breath and wiped away a tear that slipped down my cheek. "Make sure he's not alone, God," I prayed, "and, please, no emergencies tonight" . . . and began another set of hourly checks.

Judy Lawson, RN
LaCrosse, WI

A MALE NURSE ANESTHETIST

One of my favorite stories was about an event which occurred in my nursing school. You see, when I came back from Vietnam I knew I wanted to be a nurse anesthetist. For that reason I chose a nursing school connected to a hospital with a nurse anesthesia training program. That was here in Minneapolis. I did that for a purpose.

There was still a mistrust of men as nurses in the seventies. You know . . . what do we do with this guy? . . . sort of thing.

I remember my obstetrics experience. This was in a Catholic institution and they were in a quandary about what to do with me, a male student nurse who at that time was in my late twenties. Our current OB procedure in that hospital consisted of establishing a relationship with a patient who would be about 26 or 29 weeks pregnant and follow that patient through to delivery.

Everybody got their patient except me. When I inquired, the instructor said "I just don't know. I'm looking for just the right patient for you, Tom." Finally she said "I've got one for you." I don't remember the patient's name, but she was a stripper. She had decided that she wanted a child; my instructor interviewed her first and asked if she'd mind if she had a male nurse—a student male nurse—who would follow her through her last months of pregnancy. She said "Absolutely not." She was a fabulous patient and we had a great time. She had a wonderful sense of humor which made it so much easier to work as a team.

As it turned out, she was a single woman and we were talking about the birth occurring and I asked if she had an immediate family person who would be available to help her. She did have a sister but the sister and she didn't get along very well. She said "No, I'll be alone at the birth." I said "No, you can't do that. You need someone there." To which she replied "Well, why don't you be there?" I was really, really flattered and when she was admitted early one morning she told them to call me. I went over, spent most of the day with her, saw her through her delivery about seven that evening, and then went back home.

The reason I am a nurse anesthetist is because of my experiences in Vietnam in 1968 and 1969. I had worked at Portsmouth Naval hospital and had become part of an informal network of people there. One person of great importance to me was an MD anesthesiologist who had just recently received orders to go to Da Nang Naval support activity hospital at Da Nang. Just before he left I got my orders to go to Vietnam. He said "Tom, if there is anything I can do to get you into our unit at Da Nang I'll try to do that." We had a very good working relationship.

So I arrived in Vietnam in October 1968 and I happened to run into this doctor. He's retired now, living in Texas.

He was able to work it out so I was transferred to that same Da Nang hospital. My job as a corpsman there was to clean, to restock equipment, to help anesthesiologists and nurse anesthetists with patient care. It was such an experience to see the nurse anesthetist and the anesthesiologist doing what they were doing—long hours, lots of blood, sweat and tears. We came under mortar attack a couple of which will stick in my memory forever.

From time to time we were required to remove live ammunition from wounds. Literally we didn't know what would happen. At a time like that very few people were allowed in the operating room. As a gofer I had to bring in blood and run other such errands. Knock on wood. Nothing disastrous ever happened.

These were things like small grenades. I really don't know why they didn't explode when they hit the human body but our job was to remove them and save the patient.

People frequently ask if the "M*A*S*H" TV show portrayals of these events are realistic. I usually say that to me they seem to be a little romanticized.

I don't want to make a great deal of this, but when you see an eighteen year old on the surgical table, with legs blown off and other parts of the body . . . of course it is a shock.

Thanks to the people I worked with a lot of that potential shock was minimized. They were just fabulous. It was a continuously rotating staff. There were newer people and people who had been there longer. Everybody took others under their wings . . . "You know, this just happens. You can go out in back and scream and shout, but you have to come back and do your work."

Eventually I came back to the Newport Naval hospital to be discharged, I never made the war a big subject of conversation. I then worked in a hospital in Connecticut, where I had been brought up—before coming to Minnesota in 1970. I wasn't the victim of any spitting or bad treatment but, of course I didn't go down the street in uniform saying "Hey, I'm a Vietnam vet."

That was in the early seventies—that's when Vietnam, from an American point of view, got such a bad rap. There were a lot of drugs then. My brother-in-law was a medical service officer who went over in 1973. Primarily his job was to do all the drug screening for people who were coming back from Vietnam. I saw little if any drug abuse when I was there. We still had some esprit de corps, but at that time we knew why we were there. Also, those of us who were in a hospital, like I was, just didn't have time to see much of that activity.

Even though I was just a gofer, it gave me a different perspective for the rest of my life. I was about 21 when I went and I thought not about my personal safety so much—but such things as how could I leave and miss such things as "Laugh In" which was a very popular show then. How would I ever do without "Laugh In"? But I learned that life goes on and something else replaced the show, probably the friendships and camaraderie with those I worked. I learned that you have to rely on your own values a great deal, especially in that kind of situation. For that I'll be eternally grateful.

Thomas G. Healey, CRNA, MA
Minneapolis, Minnesota

ANGEL THE FROG

There is a point in every infant's development when conscious awareness begins. It's a transition from a tiny lump of living flesh to a tiny lump of living *human* flesh. I had the pleasure and privilege of sharing that precise moment with Angel the Frog.

I was on evening shift in a busy NICU (Neonatal Intensive Care Unit) when the OB (obstetrics) folks wheeled in 200 pounds of high-tech equipment cradling 900 grams of baby one winter day. A little boy had just been born 16 weeks early and, though we had the best to offer, odds were not good.

It took four of us to move him from the transport incubator to the open warmer, an open but heated infant treatment "table" on which he would stay for several weeks. I had the lightest baby load that evening and it was my turn to get the next admission, so he would be my baby.

Frail and tiny, he was hooked to every piece of equipment we had. He was intubated, warmed, cannulated and connected. No hole was left unused and a few more were added. He was X-rayed, labbed, medicated and weighed. He was assessed for actual gestation time and, sure enough, was truly only 24 weeks gestation.

His little body looked as if it were connected by skin only, every part being bendable and pliable. His face was just a little spot on a little round head, like a tennis ball with a happy face sticker attached.

The word came down the next day that his mother had named him Angel. *Angel?* A boy named Angel? Watch out, kid, Johnny Cash will write a song about you. Angel? Splayed out on his stomach he looked more like a frog to me. That's it, kid. You're Angel the Frog.

Time went by slowly for Angel the Frog. We measured blood pressure in the umbilical artery cath. We suctioned and turned. We watched his bilirubin rise and added the appropriate UV lamp. We measured urine specific gravities. We probed and touched and gave blood transfusions and lipids. One night he began to look, well, funny. His respirations were entirely dependent on the ventilator but they were, well, funny. His chest rose and fell differently. I grabbed the transilluminator, shined it on his chest and, sure enough, the whole left lung field lit up like a night baseball game. In went the chest tubes to treat the pneumothorax. A mere five cc of air ambled out through a needle between the ribs, but five cc was enough to collapse one of his lungs. Angel developed, finally, just about every complication in the book.

We had a stereo in the NICU for the staff. Played softly, it was pleasant, and helped lessen some of the background noise of beeps and buzzers that didn't signal problems. Occasionally a good Willie Nelson or Juice Newton tune would come on and someone would hum or rock a baby in time. It was nice for the nurses, and we felt that raising babies on soft country rock was good for them. Besides, we threw in a little Bach or Mozart now and again for good measure.

One evening Juice Newton was belting out her best "Break It To Me Gently." I couldn't stop myself and had to sing along to Angel. "Give me time, oh, give me time to ease the pain . . ." I was turning Angel (and all of his tubes) from his stomach to his back. "If you must go, then go slowly . . ." Suddenly, Angel's little eyelids flashed open and his eyebrows squeezed mightily together in a preemie frown. Two miniscule blue eyes crossed and wandered about the room. "Cause I'll never, never love again . . ." His eyes drifted to my face. I stopped singing and for a brief instant our eyes locked. Angel was looking at me. Not just looking, he was *seeing* me. There was a human in there somewhere. Some place in that immature brain lived a person; somebody began to inhabit that little body. "If you must go, then go slowly . . ." He focused on me again. Then his eyes drifted again and closed, retreating the little human into some secret place.

So, Angel the Frog, you like R and B music, I take it. You got it, kid. How about some good Aretha Franklin? I'll bring in a tape tomorrow.

Angel drifted down to 690 grams, the smallest person I had ever known. Aretha Franklin didn't help, though, nor did any others.

A week later it happened again. Juice was on the radio and I just had to sing. "Break it to me gently. Give me time, Oh, give me time to ease the pain . . ." I was fooling with a Razzel pump and two IV pumps which were giving me fits, (a Razzel pump was a small screw-type device which delivered the contents of a syringe as slowly as one cc/hour if desired, which was great for neonates. It's not used much any more.) I glanced down to see Angel's eyes pop wide open. Each eye went in a different direction for a moment, flashing his lovely baby blues around the room. "If you must go, then go slowly . . ." Then he saw me. He *saw* me.

Angel, dear Angel, are you in there? Look at me, kid. You've got to grow, you hear me? Stop fooling around, Angel the Frog, and put on some weight. "If you must go, then go slowly . . ." We looked at each other. Angel was not only there, he was *aware*.

He did gain weight. Weeks passed and we weaned him from the ventilator. His temperature stabilized well. He moved. He reacted to discomfort. He opened his eyes and furrowed his brow. He had a soft wail to voice his complaints. He learned to suck.

Angel's first honest meal was 2.5 cc of Similac. Not bad for a frog.

He was eventually moved to an incubator. He could be held often, and kissed, and sung to. He could be rocked and carried around the room to meet some of his nearby neighbors. And he could hear. Hear *well*. He would recognize Juice Newton from a mile away.

The rest of the staff was getting pretty tired of my singing. They referred to me as Edith Bunker on a bad day. They were not impressed.

Months passed. We placed Angel in an open crib. Angel and I were, well, soul mates, maybe. It was getting time to finish his mother's lessons on infant CPR and start learning the apnea monitor and theophyllin preparation (a device and medication to ease breathing). He was approaching six pounds now and his little face was getting fat. Also, he had developed bulges and roundness in all the right places. He even looked like a real baby now so I knew he'd be leaving soon.

One evening was going to be his last with us in NICU. He was to go home the next day. After the 11 P.M. report, I went in to say goodbye. Knock 'em dead, kid. Go out into the world and make your own music, and tell 'em you learned it from a nurse named Peggy and a singer named Juice. And never forget the first moment you were truly alive. Yes, you'll take your first step with your mother but you took your real first steps with me. I love you, Angel the Frog.

Eight months later I ran into Angel's mother near the pediatric outpatient clinics of the hospital. Her preschoolers were in tow but Angel wasn't with her. We spoke for a moment—Angel's mother and pre-mother, a close and almost sacred relationship. Of course I asked her about Angel.

"Oh," her eyes looked down to her hands. "Angel died a month ago. He was off the apnea monitor and medication. He was fine, just fine. Then, one morning, I just walked into his room . . ."

I hugged her. What do two mothers say to each other? She hugged me back. We looked into each other's eyes—her lovely ones were just like Angel's. The world became quiet for a moment. Just briefly. There were no bells. No whistles, no buzzers, no crowds, and no music. We turned and walked outside to the grass. A breeze was playing with some leaves—it must be getting to be fall, I guessed. Angel's two sisters played on the outside benches.

"I loved Angel," she said.

I know. I know.

I said goodbye and took the stairs back to the NICU. "Break it to me gently, give me time, oh give me a little time to ease the pain . . . if you must go, then go slowly, cause I'll never never love again."

I had a light load that night and it was my turn for an new admits. Another Kilogram Kid had just been born and the OB folks were wheeling him in just as I arrived. He had been born 16 weeks early and, even though we had the best there was to offer, his odds were not good . . .

Peggy Lindsay, RN, MA
Hesperia, CA

TAKING MY PEERS FOR GRANTED

Christmas season is a favorite time for nurses in a hospital. It is a season to give as well as to receive and we all anticipate the holiday with excitement and anticipation. This year in the PAU (post anesthesia unit) (in some hospitals called PAR—post anesthesia recovery) was quite different from the past.

This Christmas the nurses decided to forego their annual pollyanna in favor of buying gifts for the homeless and needy. When I presented the idea to the staff, I never thought the concept would be met with such fervor and delight. In fact, the nurses were so excited that they decided to adopt a family of four children and buy Christmas toys and some of the basic necessities for them.

Nursing care in post anesthesia unit requires careful monitoring of patients who are awakening from the effects of the anesthetic agent. Respirations, pulse and neurological status are constantly monitored. Generally it is a quiet unit as the patients slowly awaken. As a result the atmosphere in the unit is quiet, while some patients still sleep.

While the patients in the unit slept, the nurse began to divide the family into sections. Two nurses were to be responsible for buying gifts for each family member, their excitement intensifying as they planned their shopping excursion. A debate started trying to plan the appropriate gift for each person. Thoughts were on the needy when suddenly from the center of the room, from one of the stretchers, a voice was heard saying "Hey, I want to get involved too."

As fate would have it, the voice came from a successful business man who was known for his philanthropic acts. His primary nurse, embarrassed about being overheard, was cajoled by the gentleman to explain the project. He listened intently and decided to donate money to the organization for buying gifts for the needy.

As a result, the PAU nurses became minor celebrities in the hospital since this experience had never happened in the past. When the patient was returned to his room, he grabbed the telephone with as much energy as possible for one who had just had major surgery and called his son.

The nurses didn't want to push for this magnanimous gesture, being fearful that people would perceive it as a solicitation for funds. At that point they really wanted the issue to die and for the man to forget what he had overheard.

An hour later a young man arrived at the PAU door and stated that he was the patient's son who had been given instructions to bring a cashier's check for five hundred dollars to the nurses. He also mentioned that his father was grateful that the nurses had allowed him to participate in such a worthy activity.

Stunned by the man's generosity, I went to his room the next day to thank him personally for his contribution. As I shook his hand in gratitude, he said that he was the grateful one, knowing that such caring, loving nurses existed and, as a result, the world is a cozier, nicer place in which to live. As we parted, I realized that I often take my peers for granted by not giving them credit for their love, compassion and concern for their fellow man.

I am now grateful for the opportunity to tell the world that there are many generous, thoughtful people in this world, people who are not only healthcare professionals but in all walks of life. They come in all sizes and shapes and I am happy to know several of them.

These are some of the joyful realities of nursing.

Mary T. Boylston, RN
West Chester, Pennsylvania

THREE HUNDRED AND TEN POUNDS

As a male nurse I was assisting the emergency room triage nurse when Caroline, a friendly volunteer, appeared before me suddenly, breathing rapidly and obviously very disturbed.

"Keith," she gasped, "Help me! I'm in trouble."

"What is it, Caroline? Are you sick?"

"No, but I'm supposedly discharging a woman from the third floor—and I can't find a wheelchair that's big enough. Everybody is practically screaming at me and I don't know what to do."

"I don't understand. How can I help?"

"She's huge. Weighs as least 250. I've looked on every floor, every station, and can't find a chair big enough for her. She can't fit into anything."

"Let's go," I said. "I'm covered here. Let's take our biggest chair and try." All the time I was thinking that we might have to put her on a gurney to get her to the husband's car.

So off we went. When we left the elevators on the third floor, from 50 feet away the station nurse gestured negatively—meaning the chair we brought couldn't possibly handle the patient.

"Let's try this big ol' surgery chair" the station nurse said, bringing out a huge old time chariot, so big it could even be laid flat like a gurney. Why, I wondered, didn't she think of that earlier so Caroline wouldn't have been so pressured?

Then we were in the patients' room. Caroline was right. This lady was huge. Apparently calmed by the reappearance of Caroline, along with a big man, she seemed much more sedate than I had expected.

We got her into the chair but I can assure you there wasn't room for a sheet of paper between her body and the chair sides. At any moment I half expected the chair's wheels to splay out, but it was too well built to have any problems.

With Caroline assisting the husband, who followed along, I pushed the lady down a long hall to the nursing station, then along another long hall to the elevator banks. Elevator traffic was heavy so we had to wait a few minutes, a rest I was glad to grab.

This lady, I said to myself, has to weight 300 pounds. When I pushed her out of the elevator, down the long carpeted hallway, I had to lean forward, digging my toes into the carpet and putting my whole 180 pounds into the effort, glad that I had been working out regularly. Caroline couldn't have begun to handle that job. Add to that the fact that this sturdy old chair didn't have swivel front wheels, so it was almost impossible to go around corners.

Her husband brought the car to the front door while I worried about getting her out of the chair and into the car. But she insisted she could handle it, a fact I had trouble accepting, remembering that it had taken three of us upstairs to turn her around and place the chair behind her. But, when the car was in place, she arose sedately, stepped off the curb and sort of crawled into the front passenger seat, aiming that enormous derriere in slacks toward me. Then she turned and sat down, while her husband shook my hand in thanks and said "Pretty good for a gal who weighs 310, don't you think?"

I tried to straighten out my back and wondered whether I should book myself into physical therapy or call an orthopod or even a chiropractor for an appointment.

As Caroline said "How could such a sweet lady let herself get that fat?" Thank God we could try to be understanding because that lady obviously had a problem, needing any help and love we could give her.

Nurse's name withheld on request
Chicago, Illinois

ASSESSING THE PATIENT

My assignment on this particular morning in the ICU included taking care of a 57 year old Caucasian male who had a medical diagnosis of end-stage CHF (congestive heart failure). After morning report I immediately went to the patient and began making an assessment of his status. (It's important for you to know that the nurse is Afro-American.) I began the head-to-toe assessment by assessing mental status. The patient was very lethargic and required frequent tactile (touching) stimulation to keep him awake.

"Mr. M, how are you?"

"Huh?"

"How are you?"

"Okay."

"Open your eyes, Mr. M., and tell me what you see."

Barely flickering his eyes, the patient said "I see you."

"You do?"

"Yes."

"Then tell me what I look like."

"Okay," barely keeping eyes open.

"Okay, Mr. M., I'm waiting. Tell what I look like."

"You look Chinese."

Of course I laughed, softly.

"Mr. M. That's a new one on me. That is the best thing I have ever been called."

I then heard a loud roar of laughter in the ICU, which was coming from the nurses and doctors who were sitting/standing at the nurses' station. This incident took place in an ICU which was small and beds were separated by curtains. Although I was assessing the patient behind curtains, every one within 20 feet of the bed could hear every word said.

Patricia L. Brown, MSN, CCRN, CS
Hewitt, TX

COMATOSE PATIENT IS AWARE OF ENVIRONMENT

Harry was yet another victim of an accident caused by an individual who was driving while under the influence of alcohol, unfortunately an all too common reason for admission into intensive care units. He was thrown out of the back of a pickup truck by the impact of the collision. Although his seventeen year old body was relatively unscathed, he suffered significant head injuries. As a nurse in the intensive care unit, I couldn't help but wonder if another young life would be abruptly ended or, even worse, left merely to exist bereft of cognitive abilities.

Yet, as a critical care nurse, I had to suspend my preoccupation with trying to find answers as to the fairness of it all and instead transfer this energy into action. Over the days and weeks that Harry remained comatose we administered medication to reduce cerebral edema, gave him enteral tube feedings to maintain good nutritional status, changed his position frequently to prevent complications of immobility, monitored intake and output to insure adequate fluid balance, monitored his level of consciousness and supported his anxious family.

We made a point to talk to him during care procedures even though he didn't respond to this communication. Someone asked his family to bring in a small radio. We tuned it to a local pop station and left it on constantly.

Gradually Harry seemed more responsive — a grimace when he was turned, a hand moving to his face when the feeding tube was manipulated. The major breakthrough, however, was when Harry uttered his first words — "Turn off the radio."

This experience was an ironic reminder to me that one can never assume that a comatose patient is unaware of the environment. It reinforced the importance of nurturing the "mind" as well as the body.

Every nurse perceives different rewards in caring for critically ill patients day in and day out. In Harry's case, the ultimate reward was seeing him return to the intensive care unit at a later date — when he came in to thank us for saving his life.

Rose Aguilar Welch, RN, MN
Ventura, California

DO YOU REMEMBER ME?

I am presently an ICU nurse (works in Intensive Care Unit) and have worked with people for many years. I enjoy making a difference and in getting involved. These two stories are dear to me.

My first story begins with a twelve year old boy out with his friends. They were reportedly teasing an elderly, retarded man. The man was holding a large tool and began swinging it in the direction of the boys. My client got hit in the mouth. By the time the ambulance arrived, Petey's swelling had almost blocked off his airway and breathing was seriously endangered. The paramedics placed a breathing tube in his mouth to transport him to the hospital.

When I met Petey he was frightened and almost wild. I told him how important it was to allow the breathing tube to stay in his mouth until the swelling went down. I really had to struggle with him, by words, to get him to leave it alone. Then, for two weeks, Petey tolerated staying in bed, during which time he had surgery on his jaw to repair the fragmented bones and left ICU with his mouth wired closed and a residually large amount of swelling. I felt I had met the challenge of keeping that boy from self harm.

Two months later a small boy touched my arm and said "Do you remember me?" Looking at his face I couldn't place him and had to ask where we had met. Both the boy and his mother said "You were my nurse in intensive care." It was little Petey! His scars were healed; his teeth were straight and his smile was a wonderful gift for me to see.

My second story does not have a happy ending but in critical care the death of a person is not always considered a failure. I often find people from all backgrounds with whom I can identify and share their feelings. Bill was a young man who had led a tormented life. He had a serious illness as a child and his mother was devoted to helping him survive and to lead as normal a life as was possible. When Bill became a teenager he began to revolt against the rigid lifestyle required by his illness. He began drinking and using drugs which made him sick and irritable. He was so difficult to live with that he ended up living alone. During this period of living alone he developed blindness and kidney disease. Once again his family cared for him. When he was not on drugs his family had nothing but glowing comments about him but, as Bill's disease progressed, his hospital admissions became more frequent; I admitted him on more than one occasion. His mother and sister were very close and the three of us were having great difficulty dealing with all of his complications. I explained everything possible to them. I showed them how to do certain things for Bill, which they were able to do. I cried with them; I told them a joke or two on rare occasions; I told them the few words Bill had spoken when they were out of the room. I cared for each of their needs.

Bill grew worse and needed surgery. He was very weak. My

coworkers were great. They gave the family information and supported them in their decisions. Everyone was helpful, but Bill continued to deteriorate.

On the day Bill died I was there. We talked and cried and laughed together. We hugged and smiled and we were there for each other. I was glad to be there for them, although it's not always easy giving of yourself in times like that. That's what makes me appreciate life. Nursing allows me to be there for people without them even wondering why.

Lisa Kiblinger, RN, CCRN
Marietta, Georgia

NOW AND THEN

In 1967, now twenty-four years ago, nursing was exciting, if a bit confusing and dangerous to one's health. I got my first job as a new graduate in a small older hospital located close enough to Los Angeles' Harbor freeway to keep things hopping, but far enough to serve a quiet, lower-class neighborhood. The hospital was planning a new modern multistory facility, but for the time being we worked in near-quonset hut conditions. Nonetheless, I was assigned to assist the head nurse develop the hospital's first intensive care unit; I'd be the day shift staff nurse with two nurse aides. I was thrilled.

We emptied a ten-bed ward and converted it to six beds, each separated by partial walls. We painted, got new linens, bought some new desks and charts, and bought some fancy, state-of-the-art equipment. One piece of equipment was an EKG oscilloscope. God, would I ever learn to interpret what that bouncing ball means. It sure would be handy if it printed out a strip like an EKG machine, so I could study it and place it on the chart.(Besides, isn't it illegal for a nurse to diagnose an arrhythmia?)

We had our opening day. Everyone from the community, including the local politicians, came to see our new unit. Color was the word of the day: pastel sheets, kelly green transparent Bird respirators, black Ambu resuscitation bags, white bouncing balls on the deep blue oscilloscopes, bright red CPR back boards, dark green oxygen tanks, and brightly colored flowered drapes.

Suction equipment was the latest. It was a gray metal suction bottle affixed to a rolling stainless steel table. There was an indentation on the table to hold a liter of saline in a glass bottle, used to rinse the suction catheter. The new defribrillator was first class too, also affixed to a rolling table with metal wheels and an extra drawer to hold the extension cords and medications. It had an instant-on feature with a pre-set dose of 400 joules.

After all the hoopla, our first patient arrived. Martha was an eighteen-year old woman from a car accident on the freeway. She had sustained two fractures in the cervical vertebrae and a ruptured spleen. We received her directly from the operating room following a splenectomy. She also had Crutchfield tongs placed on either side of her skull with traction hanging over the head of the bed, effectively immobilizing her neck.

It was customary to place fractured neck cases on a Stryker Frame, a specialized bed to facilitate frequent turning of these long-term, immobile patients. The hospital didn't have one, so I called a rental company and asked the hospital's accounting department to write out the first week's rental check — $12.00.

We placed Martha on the Stryker, assembled the traction to her skull and neck and showed her how we'd be sandwiching her in, tying the whole thing with belts and flipping her over to her stomach. She wasn't very happy about it, but she was planning to sue the guy who ran into her on the freeway, so she said she'd go along with all these stupid treatments. It might fetch a higher settlement.

Martha had the best care we could offer.

I didn't exactly have a plan of *how* I would care for her. I would just move her toward normal, away from abnormal, and tackle each problem as it came up. She managed to present quite a number of problems too. As Martha progressed through her ten-week ICU stay, I found her to be a most peculiar person. She had a remarkable aversion to her own sputum, a supply of which her body produced in unusually large amounts. I suggested to her physician we try her on Bird treatments to loosen and thin the sputum, so she could cough it up more easily. He agreed, so I gave her six treatments a day. The Bird was a transparent plastic respirator about nine inches square, mounted on a rolling stand. As Martha inhaled the oxygen, the Bird further forced pressurized air into the lungs. We could add medications or saline to a nebulizer to be inhaled. Positive pressure—what a marvelous idea. It could even be set up to deliver controlled breaths to patients who could not breathe on their own. The Bird—what a great invention.

Martha hated it. However, she did have great plans for the settlement money. I would cajole and coax, but it was often a battle of wits. Eventually sputum would make it to her mouth, without her coughing, which she didn't like to do either. She would grab thirty or forty tissues from the extra large box on her table, force them into her mouth, retrieve the sputum and roll the tissues into a large wad. From the wad stage, the ball of tissues would unwind as she tossed it mightily onto the floor. Tissue floated like snow everywhere around her bed.

Turning Martha was also a problem. She was a thin woman and her skin was not happy with all this bed rest. After a customary explanation, followed by listening to her arguing, the nurse aide and I would finally just turn her. Each turn was accompanied by a falsetto soprano scream and a variety of comments regarding my mother's marital status at the time of my birth. Other patients in the area began clocking their medication times based on Martha's every two-hour diatribes.

Martha hated hospital food. I redesigned her diet a dozen times before we hit on food that was nutritious and suitable to her. Although I weighed her and tried to control her diet, she rapidly gained on her new diet, accompanied by some Elvis records at mealtime. Counting calories or measuring intake didn't work because too much food landed on the floor with the tissues or perhaps on the wall if it were sufficiently aerodynamic.

Ten weeks of nursing Martha was about as short as the time it took to create the solar system.

At last her cervical vertebrae healed, the traction and Crutchfield tongs were removed and we moved Martha to a standard bed. Her physician told her as soon as she could walk across the room she'd be moved to a new ward. Rehabilitation began. We had done range-of-motion and passive exercises all along, and her neuromuscular function was intact, but she insisted all fractured neck cases were too weak to walk and required years of therapy. First sitting on the edge of the bed she insisted standing or walking was absolutely out. No amount of explanation or comforting reassurance was helping.

Then I moved the box of tissue to a table about six feet away. She'd either hock it on her sheets or get out of bed.

She got out of bed.

We moved her to the ward.

Her bed didn't stay empty long. Mr. Porter, an eighty-year old Southern gentleman farmer with end-stage lung disease, was admitted in severe respiratory disease. Low-dose oxygen, positioning, medications — nothing seemed to help this man. He was struggling mightily to breathe; his skin was blue and his pulse was racing. His EKG showed a ball bouncing so fast I could only guess the rate and rhythm. Suddenly his pulse slowed and he dropped into cardiopulmonary arrest. I called a code blue. (Editor: a near-death alarm requesting immediate assistance from a selected cardiac team.) Seventeen people (seven nurses, four physicians, a pharmacist, two orderlies, a kitchen worker and two off-duty ambulance drivers), showed up to help save this man's life. During the CPR the head nurse called me aside to give report to the oncoming shift. The other would continue resuscitation. I gave report and left. My shift was over.

The next morning, however, it seemed like I had never left. I walked over to Mr. Porter to have a look before morning report. His eyes rolled back in his head and his 40-plus respirations suddenly stopped. I called out for help. Our Ambu-bag was not nearby, (Editor: An Ambu-bag is a breathing assist bag) so I pulled his head back, opened his airway and began mouth-to-mouth breathing. But his lungs were not inflating — I heard some horrible air leak. I looked down and found a tracheostomy, which had apparently been done during the night. (Editor: a tracheostomy is a surgically performed operation through the trachea to allow the patient to breathe.) Someone found the Ambu and I began Ambu-to-stoma breathing while someone else started chest compressions. We gave sodium bicarbonate. We gave epinephrine. I suctioned his tracheostomy and started to rinse the catheter in the saline bottle. The bottle was not there on the stand. Someone had knocked it over on the floor during all the commotion. My feet crunched on glass and I saw the saline run across the floor. Mr. Porter went into ventricular fibrillation so I turned on the defrillator. I yelled "Clear" and every-one stepped back. I applied the paddles to his chest and pressed the button. Mr. Porter jerked violently as the current went through him.

The machine let out a loud pop and I flew through the plate glass window behind me, grounded by the saline solution.

Mr. Porter survived the CPR.

I bled.

Three days later Mr. Porter's kidneys failed. We began peritoneal dialysis through a catheter placed in his abdomen. Procedure: run in 1500 cc's of dialysis fluid, wait fifteen minutes, draw off whatever would flow out. Run in, draw out. Over and over. Mr. Porter also had a large bleb on his lungs—a balloon-like spot about to blow out. It did and the lung collapsed. We placed a chest tube in his chest cavity to draw off the extra air. I placed the far end of the chest tube in a three-bottle, water-sealed set-up on the floor.

He arrested two more times.

Finally I asked the $64 questions of Mr. Porter's doctor. "Should we be doing all this? Does he want all this? Can his family afford all this?"

The doctor was highly incensed, or maybe a bright red face was just normal for him. "The law," he said "is very clear on this. We are required to do all in our power to save his life. You do not stop what you've begun. And you are the last person who has a right to ask that anyway. Nurses are not to be involved with this. The subject is closed."

Mr. Porter went into a coma lasting three weeks, then died. When his lovely widow received his hospital bill, she left California and was never heard from again.

The bed still didn't cool off. Thirty minutes later Roy Stedman was received from the operating room following a TURP (a transure-thral resection of the prostate). A two-way catheter from his bladder was connected on one end to a 1500 cc bottle of bladder irrigant hanging above on the IV pole. Below, on the floor, was an empty 1550 cc bottle into which was stuck the far end of a long plastic tube emptying the irrigant from the bladder. By rapidly dripping, the irrigant flowed into the bladder and back out to the collection bot-tle on the floor, carrying with it all of the blood and clots leaking from the prostatectomy incision. In and out; in and out. Blood and clots flowed down the tube to the bottle. Sometimes the bottle overflowed onto the floor. I hated TURPs. Check the patient. Check the floor.

I charted that the irrigation returns were very bloody and guesstimated the number and size of the clots drifting down the tube to the bottle. I asked Mr. Stedman's surgeon to come in a bit later to have a look. I told him I was concerned about the amount of bleeding and reviewed the intake and output sheets with him.

"What the hell is this?" he yelled. "You have charted here that the irrigation returns are bloody and contain approximately eleven one-inch clots! What the hell does *that* mean?"

"Uh, well, that's what I've been seeing. That's what's concerning me."

"How do you *know* it's blood? Did you test it? How do you *know* it's a clot? Never, but NEVER chart 'blood.' It's 'red-tinged fluid' you idiot. Nurses don't EVER diagnose blood!"

Mr. Stedman received seven units of whole blood that night and eventually stopped hemorrhaging "red-tinged fluid."

Before I realized it, a couple of decades had passed by. I didn't even see it happen. I don't remember when I last pushed around an oxygen tank or mopped up red-tinged fluid off the floor or rinsed a suction catheter in a glass bottle. I can't seem to place where I last saw a Stryker Frame, or when I first saw its replacement, a Halo traction. Patients with TURPs don't seem to bleed anymore, and we no longer stand in saline when delivering fewer joules of electricity from lower-dose, synchronizable defibrillators. I chart whatever I see, whether is it blood, sleep or behavior. I can't remember when I last wrote "Appears to be . . ." We openly ask families their feelings on the extraordinary care issue and even act as their advocates and serve on ethics committees. Computerized EKG machines print out, record and even interpret rhythms. Glass three-bottle chest tube drainage set-ups have been replaced with disposable plastic, pre-marked containers. Care plans are computerized. Birds are long gone—mega ventilators do everything but transplant a new set of lungs.

And I can't find extra large boxes of tissue anymore.

I know some nurses feel we have given away our practice, but I remember Martha and I'm grateful for respiratory therapists and their expert handling of lung and sputum-related issues. Physical therapists do range-of-motion and rehabilitate injured patients, with newer and better methods for re-walking than just moving a tissue box. Dieticians know so much more than I do about nutrition and I'm glad they're on the patient's team. Central material procures all the supplies and beds. Orth technicians, EKG technicians, phlebotomists and paramedics add more capable hands. Streamlined, four-member code blue teams instantly appear to efficiently manage cardiac arrests.

Where did all the excitement, confusion and danger go?

The only danger now is probably from communicable diseases, I guess. My greatest confusion seems only to be where nursing leaves off and other professions begin. And, yes, I guess there's still excitement, just a different kind. At least, I'm still a nurse.

I wouldn't trade Martha, Mr. Porter or Mr. Stedman for all the other jobs in the world. Either now or then.

Peggy Lindsay, RN, MA
Hesperia, California

LITTLE MIRACLES I HAVE SEEN

I have been a coronary care nurse for about 15 years now and couldn't begin to tell you of all the "little miracles" I have seen.

A woman who had witnessed her husband's cardiac arrest and the ensuing drama of a successful code, held my hand and repeated over and over again "It's a miracle, an absolute miracle."

And so it was. But such a big miracle. So orchestrated, so mechanical. Just think of all the little miracles nurses perform. Daily events, just part of the job, unheralded and unsung.

For instance:

We once had a stroke patient, totally aphasic and with some residual weakness, who was quiet and apathetic when left alone. She exuded that just-leave-me-alone-let-me-die attitude. Any attempt to care for her was a disaster. She would kick, spit, pinch, fight against medications and therapy. The staff was in physical jeopardy as they attempted hygiene and grooming.

NURSE

Her history was that of a woman who had spent most of her life in Alaska, playing honky-tonk piano in a famous saloon. No family had been located. An old clipping found in her billfold told of a presentation made by the Chamber of Commerce to a "lovely daughter of Alaska."

We were confounded by this filthy, fetid-breath animal-like person. Night sweats and unnaturally warm skin suggested an infection but she fought off examination and antibiotics with a vengeance. Social services were even contacted to investigate placement in a mental health facility.

Meal times were special nightmares. The mere sight of her dentures sent her into a frenzy. She clamped her mouth firmly closed when attempts were made to feed her pureed food but would grab avidly when offered milk or egg-nog. Obviously she was making choices so her mind seemed to be working. We became determined to find the cause of her great agitation, particularly this meal-time madness.

A number of us manhandled her into the shower and got her clean. This exhausted her and she lay quietly in bed as I began her oral care. Too tired to fight me, she allowed examination of her mouth where I found a huge abcess on the upper left alveolar ridge. She went to the hospital for oral surgery and was eventually returned to our nursing home.

Some months later I left that facility; the last I saw of her she was playing honky-tonk piano for the luncheon crowd. She was still without speech and a bit uncertain with her thumping left hand chords but very much in her glory.

At another time Marj and I were standing in the hospital lobby waiting for others to join us for an after work drink. A dapper, elderly gentleman walked slowly by, plopped himself down on a sofa and immediately fell asleep.

"Funny old guy. He sure fell asleep fast."

"Yeah. Wish I could drop off like that. Doesn't seem quite natural."

In seconds we were shouting and shaking, feeling for a pulse that wasn't there.

The receptionist called a code as we lifted him to the hard parquet and did our CPR thing. First time for me.

We both were given roses by him three days later, which just happened to be Valentine's day.

I well remember a lady who was post-op after having a hip pinning. She refused to walk because "It hurts! Oh, Gawd, how it hurts" she would yell.

She was X-rayed, pre-medicated, cajoled and scolded. Each time we put slippers on her feet and began to help her walk she would cry out again "It hurts. It hurts."

"Where does it hurt?" we repeatedly asked.

"Everywhere . . . clear down to my toes."

I removed a slipper to examine her foot where I found a badly ingrown toenail. Soon the podiatrist fixed that nail and two days later she ambulated home with no more screaming about the pain.

Little miracles. How many have nurses performed? I can see them smile because miracles are just routine, the stuff of nursing, but miracles, none-the-less.

Mary K. Erickson, RN, CCRN
Coupeville, Washington

THE DENTURES

Speaking of most memorable incidents, my most embarrassing moment occurred when I was a very new nurse working in a large hospital. I had just lost a patient and was preparing him in the bed nearest the window in this two bed room—preparing to transport his body to the morgue for the mortuary to pick him up. This may not be easy for some people to read, but a deceased person's body must go through certain procedures out of respect and care. I had never done this alone before and was naturally somewhat nervous about it.

And I was in a hurry to get him out of there and to the mortuary without disturbing the patient in the other bed who was unaware of what was going on. Anyway, I prepared his body as quickly as possible and was preparing to transport him downstairs to the morgue, when I saw his dentures in the usual cup on his bedside table. I quickly grabbed them and stuffed them into his mouth and rushed him downstairs and into a drawer.

When I returned to give normal care to his roommate, the other patient said "Miss, have you seen my teeth? I laid them on this table but can't find them now."

Good Lord! He had laid them on the deceased patient's table, the wrong table.

I thought fast, for once in my life, and said "I'm cleaning them for you, sir. I'll have them back soon."

Then I rushed downstairs to the morgue, probably taking the stairs two at a time, retrieved the dentures, and returned to my floor.

Of course I did clean and sterilize the dentures and returned them to their correct owner, thanking my lucky stars that all had worked out acceptably.

Joanne Murnane, RN
Hastings, Minnesota

ONE OF THE FIRST NURSE STEWARDESSES

I was one of the first nurse/stewardesses for Northwest Airlines. In the early days it was required by law that all stewardesses be registered nurses. And it was while I was flying in 1944 that the government came along and said "No more nurses for stewardesses because we need them all for the war effort." That is why the airlines no longer carried nurses; at this same time great effort was being made to train more nurses. Although I was at St. Mary's hospital, four floors were quickly added to the eight-story nursing dormitory at General hospital, in Minneapolis, to provide quarters for the increased crop of student nurses.

I didn't go to General hospital with the rest of my group but went to St. Mary's and let me tell you that if you took your nursing education under nuns, you became a good nurse because they were good teachers and demanded that you know what you needed to know. They were dedicated people who did their best on anything they took on.

And we were necessary on the airline. Even if it just gave the passengers some security and comfort, in the sense that there was somebody aboard who knew what to do if needed.

Yes, we were flying in the DC-3s and you are right, when they were on the ground, it was quite an uphill climb inside the airplane just to get to your seat.

I was based in Minneapolis and from there was given my trip assignments, usually to the west coast. When flying to Seattle, for example, we would change crews at Billings. Yes, this was the beginning of heavy commercial flying and we had a lot of people taking their first flights, a lot of motion sickness, and this was before anti-motion sickness medication was popularized.

Of course it was also before the airlines could go high enough to get above the choppy areas. It was frequently pretty dreadful up there.

You could see things — the trees atop the mountains, the beautiful lights of a city when you came in low — over Chicago and suburbs for example.

It reminds me of flying into Hong Kong. Last year I flew around the world on the Concorde. Coming into Hong Kong you fly through an alley of very high condominiums — your plane just glides down there and sits down right in the middle of the city. For anyone who has flown a lot, it is a very thrilling landing. Like Star-Trek.

The next day after we came into Hong Kong, the local English-language paper talked about the passengers who arrived and described us as "the rich but not very famous people." Of course that didn't make anyone feel too great.

Anyway, that was last year and this is now. I'm glad it is behind me and am very glad I made the trip.

There were two very neat women on this trip, from Maine, who had gone around the world previously, by ship, and it had taken them a month of constant traveling to make the trip.

Drinks? No, we didn't serve them. If anyone came aboard who was intoxicated, we were supposed to put them off. It still applies today but isn't enforced as much as in earlier days.

For food we first served little box lunches . . . usually a sandwich, maybe a roll, a couple of cookies and maybe an apple. We would take a pillow from the rack overhead, place it on the passenger's lap and place the box of food thereon. Later, not much later though, we had trays, which had a linen cloth and a linen napkin thereon. We would open the boxes, take out the food, place it on the tray and serve that to the passengers. That was quite an improvement.

We were pretty highly regarded as a group of people. I practically never heard that remark about being flying waitresses. So many nurses wanted to be stewardesses that it was hard to get a job. I applied constantly for two years to Northwest Airlines before I got called up, and I had good qualifications.

Everyone coming out of nursing school thought how romantic and exotic it would be to be a stewardess. And it was too. It was all so new to most of us. You can't fail to appreciate the attitude of us as young women.

We have a daughter in Edina who has been flying for 23 years. She and I were the first mother/daughter NWA stewardess combination.

I resigned from the hospital when I went on the airline job of course, but was still considered an active nurse, and still was licensed.

I met my future husband while I was a nurse and he a patient. He had virus pneumonia and was not expected to live; virus pneumonia was almost always fatal at that time. But he was one of the first patients to receive penicillin in 1940 and survived. I was his special nurse for one month which meant I spent eight hours a day with one patient. This was a somewhat common procedure for a very ill patient. Specials were always RNs, of course, not students. Soon ICU (intensive care unit) nurses replaced special care nurses in most cases. Obviously, the patient and I fell in love and were married.

When I finished my job with NWA, it was during the war and my husband was stationed in Texas; we came back to Minneapolis, had four children and in about 1965 President Kennedy said "We need nurses. I will reeducate all the nurses who used to work and we'll get the help we need." So, in 1955 I went back to Mount Sinai hospital and took the refresher course; I expected to learn something but in no way thought I'd ever go back to work.

I think the course was about three months long but, as I said, I didn't intend to work, because I hadn't worked for 25 years while I was raising my children. At St. Mary's hospital, for example, all of the heads had formerly been my contemporaries. They heard I had taken the course and said "We need nurses. Will you please give us some of your time?" I said "Well, sure, I'll give you one day a week, about three hours" and they said fine, so I started working again. That got me interested anew.

I was probably forty or so and restarting my career. But at that point when you haven't worked for so long, it's very meaningful when someone comes to you and says "Will you work for us?" instead of me going to them and applying for work. I considered it a great compliment but they needed a warm body.

Anyway, I did that for perhaps a couple of years. Then St. Mary's hospital opened its alcoholic drug treatment center. They were the first hospital in the United States to have one. I would be sent to the drug treatment area and told to wait for someone to have a drug seizure. While sitting there, hearing these comments, I thought "What am I hearing? What's going on here that I know nothing about?"

I got interested in that and attended a course at the University of Minnesota which was offering studies to people trained in other fields who wanted to be alcohol and drug counselors. I was one of their first graduates. Yes, I'm a perpetual student, even at my age. I like it.

Something I learned in counseling is that anything I do is to help myself. Anything anyone does should be to help themselves. But that's not what you usually hear. It's always that trite answer "I want to serve people, or humanity."

That's where they teach you "Hey, you're not doing that for others; you're doing it for yourself. Because you feel better after doing something for other people." It's not an easy concept to understand or to accept but it's very true. You feel good and, at the same time, the patients are benefiting from it. When I was working for Hennepin county, I had a director who was very good. She was hiring for the county and told me once that whenever she got someone who said I want to help people I stopped the interview and went on to someone else.

After I finished that course I was hired by Hennepin county so I had quite a bit of work with alcoholics. I am not an alcoholic and was one of the few who got into that area of work without being an alcoholic.

NURSE

I had the whole hospital, from the emergency room to psych wards. Lots of alcoholics. I was told that most patients in that hospital are there with alcohol-related problems. Accidents, liver damage, all these terrible things related to alcohol.

When the doctor realized that a patient's problems were caused by alcohol, he would call me. I was a referral service, really. I knew where the patient could be sent, who would pay the bills and where he might find a better life style.

I liked this work very much and they said I was good at it.

Are there many alcoholics among nurses? you ask. Not a lot but there are some who are pill users. When I was in hospitals years ago, medications were always too easily available. Now someone has to account for every single medication. So there were a lot of girls that became dependent on sleeping medications and amphetamines. Of course it's a very stressful job.

Yes, in those days we did have an assigned patient(s) load. It means so much to the patient to see her/his own nurse come on duty, to know that there is continuity of treatment. It's not so good when the patient feels he never sees the same nurse again. If that practice is changing, I think it is a big mistake.

I've had a good life. A life of very good health, for which I am thankful. Why? I came from pretty good stock. My father died a couple of years ago at 103. He was always healthy; I never remember hearing him complain. He wasn't an eater and had a very light appetite.

I like to take risks. Even if I lost my life suddenly, I've had a great life. I'm going to Yugoslavia next week with a tour group. People tell me I'm silly to take the risks of the political situation in that country. That doesn't bother me. Who's going to keep an old lady over there? They'd want to send me home anyway.

Another good thing about nursing is that it opens so many doors. For example, I married a patient.

Maxine Lapierre, RN
Minneapolis, Minnesota

FUNNIEST THING I EVER SAW

I had never seen Joe at the club before. That's an athletic club of which I'm speaking, one of a group of full-service clubs offering everything from weight training to tennis, including aerobic dancing, body building and body renovation.

The men's locker rooms of these places are, in case you haven't been around them, much like locker rooms in high schools and colleges, except for a predominance of middle-aged and elderly men. They are big places in the cities, with lots of showers, whirlpool baths, steam rooms, wash basins, plenty of deodorants, after-shave lotions, hair sprays, etc.

This particular club, unlike some others, does not furnish complimentary towels. A member either rents one for the day or brings his own in his gear bag.

Joe had apparently done neither of these things. He didn't have a towel.

I first noticed this when I saw him drying his face and hair on a roller towel, a device in the wash basin area to supplement a member's bath towel.

Now you must understand that Joe is a big man—very big. Big shoulders, big neck, big body frame. Also he had a big belly.

Then I turned from my shaving to see Joe trying to dry his back with the roller towel. It was the funniest thing I have ever seen. Here's this big man backed up to a roller towel trying to scratch his back on the elusive towel by doing something like a Latin dance, body cruising in circles, hips going laterally, and quite obviously having a hell of a time getting into contact with that lightweight towel. I turned away to keep from showing my mirth.

Later I saw him down the hall, still naked, standing in front of a huge floor fan, attempting to dry himself a little lower down with the rushing air.

You had to be there.

Now, forgive me, dear reader, but you may ask what this has to

195

do with a book about nurses. My answer—nothing. I just wanted to share this experience with you and, after all, it is my book.
William H. Hull

NINE FISHHOOKS IN ONE PERSON?

The emergency room of the community hospital in the Florida Keys received word from the Coast Guard.

"A commercial fishing vehicle has called in asking for help. They have a fisherman with nine fishhooks in his body . . . and we're going out to get him. Will be back with him in a couple of hours."

Of course we couldn't believe that any fisherman, particularly a commercial one, could manage to get nine fishhooks caught in his body. How could it happen? Who could be that awkward? That stupid?

Of course we spent the next hour making preparation. Who would do the minor surgery—nine times? Would he use a local anesthesia or would the surgeon prefer greater patient release? Would he want to cut off the shanks of the fishhooks and pull them through the rest of the way, or make incisions and remove each one individually? Lots of problems to anticipate. Was it one of the many local people whom we knew? If we knew his name we could check records for allergies and most recent tetanus booster.

But, above all, how could it happen?

With huge numbers of sport fishing people in our community, we have seen about every kind of fishing accident possible, but never—I say never—had any of us ever seen anything like nine fishhooks caught in one person's body.

We waited—and waited.

Then we had the call from the Coast Guard.

"We've got him and coming in. But it's not nine fishhooks. It's one number nine fishhook."

What a difference! The radio operator on the fishing boat had probably garbled the message so it couldn't be heard perfectly. Hence the misunderstanding.

Soon they were there with the patient and it wasn't that terrible an occasion.

The #9 fishhook is large. A photograph, actual size, is attached. It's 3¼ inches long and opens to about one inch, with a vicious barb at the end. It had caught the patient under a rib and wrapped around that rib. The patient recovered and everything turned out fine.

But nine fishhooks in one patient!

Name withheld on request.

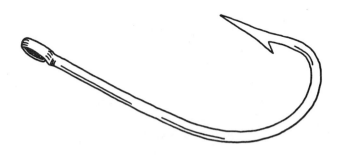

THE QUIET PARENT

I am a nurse in pediatrics in a large medical center and will carry Sammy's face, name and story with me for a very long time, maybe forever.

He is a seven-year old boy who had the misfortune of being on the bad side of a particularly nasty mule on the family farm. The injury he received when the mule's foot met his head left him with a skull fracture which the neurosurgeon described as being a "jigsaw puzzle of slivers," brain lacerations, contusions and profound cerebral edema (swelling).

Sammy had spent days in the pediatric intensive care unit s/p craniotomy (*status post* craniotomy simply shows that the patient had undergone a surgical opening of the skull) and repair of his injury, being ventilator dependent much of that time. He was transferred to the floor at the end of my shift Friday with a Keofeed tube in place and a horseshoe-shaped incision on the right side of his head. Like most head injury patients, he was extremely combative and needed constant restraints to prevent injury to himself, or dislodgement of his tube. "Great weekend ahead," I thought to myself, grimly eyeing this latest addition to an already busy group of patients.

Unfortunately for Sammy and his family, the damage done to his brain tissue was extensive. The physician had told his parents that the best they could hope for was a child who could take food orally — but he would never walk or talk; he would always be completely dependent on them.

Saturday morning began auspiciously enough. As I made walking rounds with the 11 PM to 7 AM nurse, we found Sammy's mother already dressed, knitting quietly at his bedside. Sammy had somehow wiggled out of his restraints and had pulled out his Keofeed, which lay next to him in bed. "Nice start," I thought to myself, confirming my fear of what the weekend would hold. This particular religious group are a quiet, reserved sect, not given to emotional outbursts. Although I feel I usually handle parents well, particularly in times of crisis, I found it difficult to spend any extra time in Sammy's room, not because of him, but because of the quiet, accepting, waiting manner of his mother. Having a daughter myself, I found it difficult to reconcile her seemingly passive acceptance of their tragedy and what I was positive would have been certifiable lunacy on my part had I been in her shoes.

Except for the predictable diarrhea so common in patients with bolus nasogastric tube feeding, Saturday passed without further incident. Sammy's mother did much of his care, changing his diaper, bathing him, helping me turn him without letting his free hand grab his tube. Her touch was always gentle and loving, but her quietness continued to disturb me.

Sunday started better. Sammy's mother explained that the family would be going to church but that Sammy's older sister would stay with him. She explained that the sister spoke Dutch and English and would be able to translate if Sammy needed anything. The fact that he had not made an intelligible sound in any language since his accident did not seem to figure into her thinking.

Just after lunch the call light over Sammy's door went on. The voice of his sister over the intercom confirmed my worst fear— "Sammy pulled out his tube." As I walked to his room, I mentally tallied the people who might be available to help hold him while the resident replaced the Keofeed and during the subsequent X-ray to check tube placement. In his room it was just as I had anticipated. The tube lay in his bed and his sister was vainly trying to prevent him from shredding his diaper—a lost cause.

I talked to him as I began to untie his remaining restraints and to change his diaper. What I said is not important. Probably something trivial, like "Sammy, what are we going to do with you?" But as I spoke, I looked at him and felt for the first time since I had been caring for him that he was looking at me—not the vacant wild-eyes look I had grown accustomed to, but an understanding "with-it" gaze I had not seen previously on his face.

I thought about the standing order on his chart—"May try oral fluids." We had all laughed about that. Sammy had no swallow or gag reflex at all. As I looked at him, remembering the struggles of replacing the tube the previous day, I thought, "Why not? Let's give it a try." I told his sister I was going to try to give him a drink by mouth. She looked skeptical but did not say anything. I cranked up his bed, left his restraints hanging at the sides and filled a cup with water from the sink. I cannot describe the feeling that came over me as that child gulped down 60 cc of plain old tap water—the fluttering in my stomach, the pounding of my heart, the shortness of breath. And when I went to refill the cup, Sammy spoke.

Even if I could pronounce or understand what he said, I could not reproduce it here, because he spoke in Dutch. But even to my ignorant ear, it was evident this seven-year old was demanding something. His sister's eyes opened wide as she looked from him to me and said, "He would rather have iced tea." To this day I think I flew to the kitchen to get Sammy his iced tea. After an additional 150 cc went down without incident, I decided he was ready to advance. I called his resident to ask if he could have some ice cream. I am reasonably sure the resident thought I had lost my mind or was chemically impaired. They all knew Sammy had still been a "neurologic nothing" on morning rounds. But the resident said I could try.

"Just don't let him aspirate: he goes to Elizabethtown rehab tomorrow."

I returned to my patient's room and unthinkingly asked his sister if vanilla would be all right. I was only two steps up the hall when she came after me. "He says he would rather have chocolate." It was only a short time after that when Sammy's family returned from church. In that time I was thrilled at the progress he had made, even walking to the bathroom with minimal assistance to void in the toilet. I wondered how his mother would react when she returned.

Not only his parents but his grandparents, siblings, aunts and uncles came to see him that day. They never lifted their reserve as Sammy's grandfather said "This is God's way." But the excitement in the room was palpable. And the two tears that glistened on his mother's cheeks when Sammy spoke to her in Dutch told me that, inside, she was shouting her joy from every rooftop.

The conclusion to his story is that several weeks later, after a stay at the rehabilitation center, Sammy came back to see me, walking, talking Dutch with his family and shy as many seven-year olds are with people they don't know that well. His mother thanked me for the care he had received and said how wonderful the doctors and nurses had all been. Her praise made me feel more than a little ashamed. After all, we were the ones who had pooh-poohed the oral fluid order. I had mentally cringed at the idea of letting Sammy's sister be at his bedside as an interpreter because we all "knew" he would never speak again. But these people with their quiet faith, despite what must have been a terrible heartache for them, had believed in their God, in Sammy, and in us.

The significance of this event in my professional life is multifaceted. First, it made me examine myself and the way I deal with others, particularly the quiet parent. Even though it may be uncomfortable I make myself take extra time to talk to that quiet mom or dad. Often that reserve is a facade for their inner terror. Although they appear to be coping, a few gentle questions about the kids at home, their jobs, or some trivial chitchat can open them up, allowing them to express fears, thoughts and questions.

The second area of significance has to do with labels. Although we are taught as nursing students that labels such as "slow" or "retarded" can become self-fulfilling prophecies, I do not think that concept fully impacted on me until that day. Now, even though I do not always succeed, I make the extra effort to feed a baby orally when a gastrostomy tube looms in her future, or try extra hard to teach a mom who has difficulty grasping the importance of medical therapy for her child. Labels, as I found out, can be misleading and can dull good nursing sense.

Finally, this event is most significant because I regard it as something of a miracle. Having worked on pediatrics for six years, I know physicians give the parents an optimistic but realistic prognosis if possible. To hear their pronouncement for Sammy signified that this was indeed a sad situation. I have since heard other parents talk about their "miracle baby" or the miracle that happened to their child and I have to think there is an intangible something in human beings. Perhaps it is faith in the God of their choice or the essence of the human spirit, an inner drive without obvious source. This is what keeps me at this difficult, wonderful job—helping these children physically, hoping that their miracle will come through for them. On those long days when every IV is blown and every resident is in a foul mood, the miracle and triumph of Sammy can still make me smile.

Kimberly Baird, RN, BS
Lebanon, Pennsylvania

TAPE DOWN MY PILLOW

It was my first day on the job and I was helping care for an elderly man, truly an old curmudgeon.

He was crabby, complaining of everything and anything. As demanding as anyone could be, he would talk about nothing except his money and financial worth. Later I realized that he was probably scared of the likelihood of death and didn't want to face the unknown. He did keep indicating he didn't know what to do about his money, if and when . . .

He called me in and asked me to tape his pillow.

"Tape your pillow?" I asked. "What do you mean, sir? I've never done that before."

"Well," he retorted, "are you so green you don't know anything? Just tape it so it'll stay in one place."

So I got some 3M Transpore tape and taped his pillow horizontally and vertically. I taped it to the sheet and I taped it to the head of the bed. I'll bet I used a whole role of tape and he still wasn't satisfied.

"Tape it some more," he yelled. "Really get it held down. You don't know nothing. Didn't they teach you anything?"

I wanted to say that this was my first day on the job and that maybe that wasn't taught until the senior year. But, of course I kept my mouth shut.

So he seemed satisfied and lay back on the pillow, moving around some before settling down and going to sleep. Ahha, I thought. I finally satisfied him.

But I was wrong. So very wrong. Soon his call button lit up and I went running.

"Get me out of this thing," he yelled. "It's got me a captive."

Then I saw it. He had moved his head around enough that some of the tape had been turned over, sticky side up, and his hair had matted into the tape.

Naturally I wanted to burst out laughing but didn't dare do it. I wanted to explode, if not in hilarity, then in anger with a cutting remark "Well, you old fool, you had to have it this way." But, no, that would be a real no-no.

So I just helped him untangle from the pillow, straightened the bed and left him for a night's sleep . . . and broke up out in the hall.

I wasn't on shift the next day but when I returned the following day I headed straight for his room. I wanted to see how the other shifts had handled him.

Well, what do you know. No tape in sight. Someone had either told him off or he had not made his demands again.

I thank God that there haven't been many patients that difficult to please. Most are concerned and happy about any attention we can give them—and we do try very hard.

Adeline Hardy, NA
Minnetonka, MN

THE PROUDEST MOMENT OF
MY NURSING CAREER

I've been a registered nurse for 4½ years now, all of which has been in the surgical ICU department of a 524 bed hospital. I've always enjoyed the work I do, caring primarily for post-operative heart patients. However, my most memorable moments as a nurse come from my experience when the National Guard unit to which I belong was called up for duty in the Persian Gulf.

Our unit, the 17th Evacuation Hospital, was located approximately 30 miles west of Hafu Al Batin, Saudi Arabia, and some 20 miles south of Iraq. We were supporting soldiers of the VII corps, who spearheaded a flanking maneuver into southern Iraq on a search and destroy mission against the Republican Guard.

Fortunately the number of casualties was quite low. Nevertheless, we saw the horrible effects of war. We saw it in the faces and bodies, and heard it in the voices of the soldiers we cared for. There is nothing glamorous about war.

The surgical ICU where I was working cared for a number of brave Americans who sustained serious combat injuries. I was very proud to do the best that I was able for these real heroes. I have memories of all those I cared for, but one moment stands above the rest. It is by far my proudest moment as a nurse.

We received a patient from surgery who had stepped on a land mine. Both of Russell's legs were shattered; his right hand, abdomen and chest had received multiple shrapnel injuries, as well as his right eye. I cared for Russ over a stretch of three 12-hour shifts. He initially was on the ventilator immediately following post-op. He did well and was extubated the following morning. As with all of our combat injured patients, early psychological intervention was as critical as their physical needs. Battle fatigue was obvious. Concerns of injuries and fears of long term results are immediate. Family members are on their minds; have they been contacted? How are they coping with it? They are also interested in the welfare of their comrades. Over the next two days Russ and I covered all these concerns and more, as well as caring for his physical injuries.

Russ recovered well and on the day we evacuated him to Germany our hospital commander awarded him the Purple Heart. I was at his bedside when he received the medal. Russ, quite ill and weak, managed to raise his badly injured right arm to a salute and say "I love my country." Tears still come to my eyes when I think of that moment, for it is the proudest moment of my nursing career. I know I did my best for this brave American who carried out the ultimate act of patriotism by putting his life on the line for this country we all love.

Another memorable experience of the Gulf war comes from caring for David who received serious injuries injuries to both thighs, scrotum, an index finger—all occuring when the Bradley fighting vehicle he was riding took a hit from an Iraqui tank. Despite his injuries, David was able to provide first aid to surviving crew members (two were killed), to set up a fighting position, to call in for assistance, while the vehicle and crew were under heavy enemy fire.

When help arrived David was found attempting to save a machine gun from the wrecked vehicle. He told the medics to care for the other crew members first.

David told me his story which I recorded in my diary in early March. That story appears in "Stars and Stripes" soon and later in "People" magazine, wherein he was highly praised. He's also been nominated for a Silver Star. It's a great feeling to know I provided nursing care for this courageous young man.

Thank God for soldiers like Russ and David.

John T. Specht, RN
Marshfield, WI

THE CUTTING EDGE OF NURSING

Feeling the burnout begin after one particularly rough time on the unit, I sat back with a drink in my hand and my dog in my lap, wondering where I'd gone wrong. My intentions were good. I always cared about humanity—our disease, our suffering. And the human body hadn't changed in my years of nursing. Technology (the T-word) had certainly exploded. (Ever notice that the fellow who invents technology is never there to trouble-shoot or monitor the thing?) I wanted to be a good nurse. I just never figured all the new what-its and do-dads would be invented, nor did I realize I'd be crawling over them to reach my patient. I had heard the cutting edge of nursing was in the T-word . . . somewhere. All I ever really wanted to do was to ease suffering. I never planned on the beeps, bells and whistles.

Taking my usual doses of depression and low self-esteem (two of the major food groups, coffee and fast food being the other two), I decided to find a new direction in my nursing career. Where was nursing going to be in 10 or 20 years? What would nursing care look like and what would I be doing? I decided to find the true cutting edge of nursing, point myself in that direction and prepare for the future. The present was getting to be a lot of hard work. I needed the excitement of the hunt—the anticipation of self-discovery. I took three aspirin. I knew I was up to this.

I went back to school. All nurses in burnout go back to school. Some actually survive it. I studied mega-issues that drive the clinical arena, like science and knowledge bases, autonomy, regulation, cost-cutting, professionalism, marketing, computerization, accountability and the application of political pressure in health care. I got a good dose of the future. With issues like these, my quarry had to be in there somewhere. In spite of studying hard it just wasn't clear enough to me. I searched but I couldn't find the cutting edge. Maybe I'm not smart enough to see it.

What I did find was money. Money, rolling out of my pocket. The college brochure says the cost of a class is $395, and I can use that as a tax write-off if I work it right. What I couldn't write off were the parking costs (and two parking tickets), the study sessions requiring lots of coffee and snacks, new brakes on my car, the tendonitis in my left shoulder from carrying books around, and the newspaper ads to find a small collection of decent babysitters. (My kids started calling me "the lady who changes the sheets every week.") I earned my M.B.A.—Motherhood by Absentia. Nine thousand dollars later I was smarter.

My salary was the same when I got back to work. Surely the cutting edge of nursing would now be obvious to me. I worked in a unit filled to the brim with the T-word. However, the building had not kept pace, so much of the T-word items required extension cords across the floor. When the patient looked funny, I didn't check the patient. I checked the plugs. When patients needed attention down in Cat-scan I went. When the medications were needed STAT, I went to Pharmacy to pick them up. I paged physicians to tell them another physician wanted to consult. "What for?" they'd ask. Half the time I never knew. I did EKGs on weekends because the technicians were off. I put little yellow stickers on 5x7 cards. I microwaved TV dinners for hungry new mothers who delivered in the night. I taught an intern how to do a Dubowitz on an infant. I taught new grads how to start IVs and counselled them on interdepartmental relationships and cafeteria food. I drew STAT blood work because the lab only made rounds at certain times. I checked unused, always-locked crash carts.

I held a 10 year old boy in my arms as he died because his parents weren't there. It seems he was declared brain-dead and was to be an organ donor, so his parents grieved and left. He was brain-dead but not exactly mortuary-dead. I got the mortuary-dead end of it, which apparently doesn't count. Death was recorded when he was declared brain-dead. I didn't know how to chart all the nursing care I gave him between the brain-dead and the mortuary-dead times.

Patients seemed so much sicker. The issues seemed so much more clouded. If the cutting edcge of nursing were on this unit, I wasn't finding it. I probably wasn't looking hard enough. Maybe I'm not perceptive enough.

I went to seminars at over-priced hotels. I got bloated from the restaurant food, to the tune of about three pounds per seminar. I subscribed to nursing journals reporting complicated information I didn't even realize I needed to know. I joined professional associations that discussed everything from the pluralities of nursing theory to the latest changes in licensing fees. I wrote a lot of checks for membership dues; one year my professional memberships cost me more than my car insurance. I sought others' opinions. I got everything from "Documentation! That is the cutting edge of nursing in the next century," to "Benefits—nursing will go nowhere without better benefits!"

My search was not going well. I was losing hope. Maybe I wasn't sophisticated enough. Then a friend, Marie, called me late one night. Funny how fate works. Always after you've spent your life savings, you've got 110,000 miles on your car, and your husband says "Not another headache?" It seems my friend's mother had been ill. Could I come over to their house? I thought about it a minute. Here I was in the midst of all this exciting self-discovery and she wants me to look at her mom. She's got to be kidding. "OK," I told her, "but don't expect miracles. She probably belongs in a hospital."

I met Mrs. Davis in her home. She's just had a CVA. Right hemiplegia, aphasia, urinary cath, constipation, and in a wheelchair (she weighed too much to lift alone). Oh, Lord. This lady belongs in at least an extended care hospital. Marie told me that her mom had a little money—only Medicare—and that there were no long term beds available within an 80 mile radius. There was no place for her to go but home. There was a home health team available, but not for several days, and the cost was high. Marie asked if I could help. I sat in the chair and lit a cigarette. Yes, I still smoked.

I pondered Mrs. Davis's case. She had many difficulties, but the least of which were all the potential problems that could arise from such a sedentary condition. She needed help with eating, toileting and all movements. She was depressed and frustrated. Her mealtimes consisted of being fed baby food by her daughter while in her wheelchair in front of the television; everyone else ate at the kitchen table. It was a major tactical effort getting her into bed at night and seeing to her other comforts—and listening to her sobs in the dark.

I did not need this. Give me the unit with too much T-word, extension cords, and little yellow stickers. Mrs. Davis was going to be a lot of work. "Okay, Marie, I'll try. But get your entire family over here. We have to talk." After all, I rationalized, I am a friend and a nurse. Overextending is what we do best.

The family arrived. They were a supportive group, if not intensely knowledgeable about health matters. We examined Mrs. Davis together. We talked at length. "Okay," I said, "here's what we have to do." I gave them lists of the top items to tackle first; I made lists of interventions with how-to instructions; I drew pictures and made lists of phone numbers; I instructed in medication regime. We talked late into the night about giving it all you've got, even when you are tired and progress is slow. I told them I would visit every three days.

I left that night, thinking this family is going to have to pull together and take over. There's only one of me and lots of them. Since when do I owe this to humanity? Nurses quit doing this stuff fifty years ago with the invention of real hospitals.

I did visit her every three days. Periodically her needs changed and she'd make a little progress, so I changed the top four priorities. I rewrote instructions and taught the family everything from bladder training to lifting techniques. It was a lot of work, especially on top of my full time job and teaching the kids the value of cleaning their rooms at least twice a year. As time passed, Mrs. Davis started to perk up. She began speaking fairly clearly in sentences. She fed herself. She was beginning to move herself safely from the bed to the chair and back again. She was on her way.

I guess I was just overwhelmed at work and too tired to continue my self-discovery of the cutting edge of nursing. I only came into nursing to help people cope with difficulties associated with illness. I wanted to provide comfort, security, protection and disease prevention. I wanted my sharp eye to detect subtle changes in behavior, reactions and signs. I didn't come into all of this to find any cutting edges of anything anyway.

It's been a year now since I met Mrs. Davis. She thinks I'm the tops. Life at her home is better now, even though she worries constantly about future health expenses on a fixed income. My bank account is recovering and my kids can remember my name. My disposition is so much better that my husband thinks I take hormones.

I never did find the cutting edge of nursing in the 21st century.
Peggy Lindsay, RN, MA
Hesperia, California

Reprinted by special permission from MODERN NURSE magazine

O.R. NURSE AND PATIENT
BECOME FRIENDS

An operating room nurse is both a clinical and a technical nurse. Both aspects are equally important in providing quality nursing care within the operating room setting. The following exemplar concentrates more on the clinical aspect of O.R. nursing.

It was the day before Thanksgiving; the schedule was busy for this time of the year. Mrs. Panetelli had just been brought over from Day Surgery and was waiting in the holding room, to be assessed before going into the O.R. She was scheduled for a mediastinoscopy —surgery in the median dividing wall of the thoracic cavity. She was in her late forties, a wife and mother of several children. I approached her stretcher, confirmed her identity and introduced myself as the nurse who would be with her during her entire stay in the operating room. She appeared extremely anxious. She'd had a mastectomy two years previously for cancer and the doctors were concerned that there might be further involvement. At this moment one of the surgeons was going to take a biopsy of the lymph node.

An operating room nurse has a very short time to develop a good rapport with the patient, one of trust when the patient will know the nurse is her advocate in the O.R. I asked Mrs. Panetelli the routine but pertinent questions.

Do you have allergies? When did you last eat or drink? Do you understand the procedure that is going to be performed?

I briefly explained the procedure and what to expect once we were in the operating room. I watched her body language and facial expressions to sense how much information she wanted to know. Some patients don't feel comfortable knowing every detail about the procedure because they are already very nervous. She said she had no more questions but just lay there wringing her hands. I touched her shoulder and said "We'll take good care of you, Mrs. Panetelli. I will try to tell you everything we will be doing beforehand, so there will be no surprises. I will check to be sure your room is ready and I will take you down to it." She nodded in agreement, saying "I just want to get it over with."

I checked the chart for the necessary data, lab values, consents, X-rays, etc. We then proceeded into the O.R. Once we were in there, and masked, we only have our eyes, voice and touch to help alleviate the fear some patients feel. Mrs. Panetelli was having a local with anesthesia on stand-by if needed.

She was positioned on the table. I placed a pillow under her knees to help prevent back discomfort and adjusted the arm boards. A patient can feel helpless and vulnerable with their legs and arms strapped down, so I again explained what everything was and that it is routine and necessary for all these procedures. She was prepped, then draped for the procedure and xylocaine was injected. The surgery was underway.

During the surgery I held her hand and talked to her, trying to keep her mind off the activities around her. Occasionally she would ask what was going on. I told her and asked repeatedly if she were comfortable. This was one of those times the paperwork could wait. I wrote down the pertinent data but I felt she needed my moral support. The specimen was removed and sent to pathology for a frozen section.

We became quite friendly. Mrs. Panetelli was preoccupied with the findings and kept insisting "I know I have cancer. You'll tell me won't you, doctor?" He replied that he didn't know anything yet but would tell her when he did.

The report came back positive for carcinoma. She had cancer.

Only the doctor, the scrub nurses, and I knew what the report said. The doctor motioned not to say anything but it was difficult to hide my emotions from her because we had established such a good relationship. I wanted to tell her, to be there for support, but I couldn't.

Once surgery was over we headed back for the Day Surgery. She was crying, believing bad news was inevitable. I held her hand, trying to reassure her, telling her to wait for the doctor to give her the news.

I gave my report to the nurse, finished writing the circulating sheet and then wished Mrs. Panetelli my best. I had to return to surgery where another patient awaited me. I wanted so badly to help her when she received the news, but it was no longer my place.

I was angry at the surgeon for not telling her but he did explain to me later that he didn't know her and felt the family physician would know her better and thus know which approach to use in telling her the news.

I think of her often and wonder how she is. I hope she does not feel I betrayed her. Relationships in the O.R. are short term; it can be emotionally difficult at times.

Patricia Power, RN, CN
Wilmington, Massachusetts

FORCED INTO SURGERY

I went to work that Saturday as I always do, with mild anticipation, but without great expectations of what the day would hold. I poured my cup of ambition with caffeine and sat down to report.

Mr. S. was admitted to the hospital with throat cancer with metastasis (shifting of the disease from one part of the body to another part/s) and needed a gastrostomy tube (an artificial opening into the stomach) for feeding and nutritional support, because swallowing had become painful and difficult. He underwent this procedure on Friday. His surgeon, anticipating possible complications, spoke with him and his family regarding airway concerns since he would need to be intubated (to insert a tube) for his anesthesia and his throat was already a problem. The family also discussed with the surgeon that if he had any respiratory difficulties during his surgery a tracheostomy (making an opening into the windpipe) would be performed. Mechanically this would be more comfortable and guarantee a patent airway.

Mr. S. had his gastrostomy tube placed and with the great skill of his anesthesiologist was able to have an endotracheal tube (within the tracheal) placed orally to provide safe and comfortable anesthesia for his surgery. He proceeded to the recovery room where he was extubated and returned to his room for his post-operative course. That evening he suffered some severe respiratory distress. Fortunately, his surgeon was seeing another patient at this time and was able to see Mr. S. immediately. The surgeon was acutely aware of the circumstances surrounding Mr. S.'s difficult intubation and previous discussion with his family regarding possible tracheostomy. After attempting unsuccessfully to reach his primary physician and the patient's family, the surgeon performed an emergency tracheostomy at the bedside to save Mr. S.'s life. He was placed on mechanical ventilation and transferred to the intensive care unit. The surgeon still was unable to reach Mr. S.'s family that night and was in first thing Saturday morning to try again.

I began my usual assessment and care for Mr. S., including his level of consciousness and orientation. Yes, he was awake, alert and oriented and, yes, he did remember what happened to him and how he got here. I couldn't help but notice the sad, forlorn look in his eyes. I proceeded to explain the ventilator, its alarm, and his environment, to allay his anxiety—but his expression never changed. We continued getting to know each other and I kept performing my nursing obligations—vital signs, medications, etc. Finally I said to him "I know all of this is frightening and you seem upset. Is there anything I can do to help with this?" He looked away.

The day continued and I tried to give Mr. S. as much control over his care as possible. Finally his daughter came in. She had not yet spoken to the surgeon and she was quite alarmed to find her father in intensive care. I assured her that he was okay and that the doctor had been trying to reach her. I paged the doctor but naturally she wanted to see her father immediately. So I reviewed briefly what had happened and his current circumstances. She went into her father's room and he would not speak to her, nor maintain any eye contact. The daughter told me she was calling her brothers, there being five children in the family. As she went out to make her calls I said to her "Your father seems very upset." It was then that the daughter shared with me "He didn't want this surgery. We forced him into it."

Next, two of his sons came to see him. Same response. He looked at them with despair in his eyes, then looked away.

This family is in crisis, I thought, and no one is coping well.

I spent some time with the daughter in the waiting area where she told me that Mr. S.'s wife died of cancer about three years ago after going through vigorous chemotherapy and radiation therapy.

Mr. S. refused both of these in his case because he did not want to go through what his wife had endured. "He has been depressed since she died but after we all talked with him, he agreed to have this surgery," she said.

I spent the rest of the day getting to know Mr. S. I made it a point not to push him or discuss all that I knew; I just wanted him to trust me. Saturday night I went home but didn't sleep all that well. I could just see that despairing look.

Sunday morning I went into his room. "Good morning, Mr. S. How are you today?" He had changed very little. I knew in my heart this situation was intolerable to him and I felt his family dynamics were not assisting him in his dilemma. I said "I want you to tell me if I am wrong, but I get the impression that you object to this machine, the respirator. Is this correct? He looked straight into my eyes and shook his head affirmatively. I said "You need to tell your family how you feel. I'm sure they don't want anything to happen to you but I don't think they would want you to be forced into something you feel strongly against." He had tears in his eyes and so did I.

"We are here to help you. Would you talk to your family about this if I were here to help you?" I asked. He shook his head yes again. I related this conversation to his surgeon and to his daughter. When his family arrived his son was very angry. He said to me "Why did he talk to you?" I reassured him that it was easier for his father to talk to me because he was not as emotionally close to me as he was to his children. Nothing was decided that day but they were beginning to talk to one another. I set up a meeting on Monday with his primary physician, his family, and his surgeon. At that meeting it was decided he would be weaned off the ventilator and should he have any difficulty he would *not* be placed on mechanical ventilation again.

I went home emotionally exhausted and slept soundly.

The order to "Do Not Resuscitate" is at times controversial, emotional, but never one that is taken lightly. I have helped some family members struggle with this; usually the patient is too sick or incapable of making this decision for himself. It is not a nursing role to initiate this order, but it is a nursing role to facilitate the process. As a critical care nurse, I am trained in and perform many technical and lifesaving tasks. Technology is rapidly changing from computerized cardiac output machines to laser oxygen saturation monitors. No technology will ever replace the need for human touch and understanding.

M. Debbie Tustin, RN
Winchester, MA

I LOVED THE PRECISION OF SURGERY

Memory does play tricks and occasionally fails totally. Many of my vivid memories involve situations which are clearly not for publication—unless one were writing for the tabloids.

As to assigned patient loads, yes we certainly had them. Always too many. Never enough time to do all one would like to do. The basic care was always adequate, however, from a medical standpoint. Since student nurses constituted the bulk of the nursing staff during the war years (World War II), we brought an attitude of freshness and enthusiasm to our duties, not necessarily prevalent in other nurses. After a time in the profession one slowly comes to realize the limits of what can be done and the youthful attitude of "I'm part of the team and we can do anything" tends to abate.

Because of the war and also the financial limits of a city hospital, it seemed that we were chronically short of supplies. For instance, we nurses would rush to get sheets first thing in the morning because by mid-morning the laundry shelves were bare. Somehow, we always managed to keep the incontinent patients dry even if it meant that someone less helpless had to wait a day for a linen change. Lying in a wet bed causes the skin to break down and a bed sore to develop, which is a rather shameful event for a nursing staff.

When I rotated to a local tuberculosis sanitorium there was a disturbing event one day. Several years earlier I had an adolescent "crush" on a young man in our neighborhood. On the day I was assigned to the treatment room it was a shock to find that our patient was this same young man. He had advanced tuberculosis and was there to have pneumo-thorax procedure, an injection of air into the lung to collapse the most severely impaired lung. The remaining lung was adequate to supply him with the necessary air. The staff was dressed for surgery with masks, etc. I was shocked to see him as a patient and felt great sympathy because he was obviously extremely ill. In those days there seemed to be shame connected with TB and because of great public fear of it, the subject was generally taboo. For those reasons I did not reveal that I knew him.

It was always very easy for me to slip from the mental mode in which a patient was a "person" and into the mode where I was part of a team working on a problem. Some doctors and nurses have to learn that shift to preserve their mental health, but for me it came easily.

One of the most frustrating things I have encountered is the patient who will not comply with or refuses treatments. There was never enough time to coax or convince the patient and every episode left me with a bad feeling. This may have been one of the reasons I opted for work in operating rooms. There the patients were either asleep or, if awake, were present willingly and cooperatively.

Nurses' training is rather a blur for me because it was so long ago. But I have many memories of the operating rooms. It was often exciting there, wonderful in the truest sense, even astounding. There were the women bleeding to death from an ectopic pregnancy, who had lost their ashen pallor and began to regain normal color less than five minutes after surgery began. There were two women within the same week who had severe post partum (after childbirth) bleeding and were brought to surgery. One of them "died" on the table but was resuscitated without any of today's assisting machines —and both of those patients' obstetrical problems were solved.

There was the time a good friend was brought in with her unborn baby in distress. I was privileged to scrub on that Caeserean section—scared out of my wits at the surgeon who was known as a tyrant. I had perfect faith that he would succeed and he did. From the time the mother was asleep he delivered the baby in only forty-five seconds! I still get shivers when I think of it. Proud to be a nurse? No, make it *grateful*. . . .

Then there was the amusing and unlikely coincidence of scrubbing on both Caesereans two years apart for the wife of a famous baseball hero, and the fun of seeing the large family's joyous reaction both times.

There were less happy times, of course. It was a neverending marvel to see the beautiful, anatomical arrangement in an open abdomen or the wonder of watching a surgeon place the tip of an instrument into an area hidden from view and locating the exact nerve or duct he sought. At the other end of the scale were those cases so totally shocking at first view because of profound illness or accident, when virtually nothing could be easily identified. Those seemed to be the night emergencies and could go on for eight hours or more. Professionals who do emergency work are probably experiencing emotional highs and lows to an extreme degree seldom found in other fields.

Would I rather have been an MD? No! I'm not suited for it. I prefer working as part of a team. Physicians must make most of the decisions and carry the principal load of responsibility. This simply does not appeal to me, even though I am vitally interested in the disease process, in anatomy, physiology, and all things concerning health. On a lighter note: having watched the zombie-like interns and residents going about their business after thirty hours on duty at least twice a week, I'm sure I couldn't have done it.

Caring for needles was always a regular chore in the operating room. Floor nurses had their needles all cared for in Central Supply but we did our own in OR. Every needle was washed, disinfected, inspected for sharpness, had barbs removed and sharpness restored on a small whetstone, tested for sturdiness when attached to the hub, packaged and sterilized for re-use. It was dull and tedious work but if working with someone else, many pleasant conversations ensued.

We hated the disposable paper gowns and drapes when they first came into use but had to bow to progress. To our horror, we quickly learned that progress did not necessarily mean improvement. (Reminds me of Bill Hull's often quoted remark that "All change is not progress.")

Anyway, the paper material was certainly waterproof as claimed but one day, after a long procedure, the surgeon removed his gown to find a good deal of blood on his front. This was an open invitation to infection for the patient but, thanks to antibiotics, there was no bad result. Then we began to use a sterile square of absolutely impermeable plastic over the surgeon's mid section where it would normally touch the surgery area. This worked very well but added to the costs. I'm sure the problem with gowns has now long been solved.

I've certainly had many opportunities to use my knowledge and to practice nursing on my family—my three children, friends and acquaintances. Many times I've been able to help sort out someone's uncertainties about whether to see the doctor, and to offer support and assurance during a long-term problem.

I'm very proud to have been a nurse for most of my life.

Virginia W. Purdy, RN
Minneapolis, MN

WHAD HE SAY?

My patient lay in bed while her physician gave her the prognosis of her disease. He was saying . . .

"Well, my dear, you might just have an ulcer. First we'll place an NG tube to low constant. You'll be NPO of course. We'll keep an IV going and in the AM we'll do a GI series. Then we'll plan an upper GI the next day, and perhaps a BE. If those tests don't show us anything, we'll do an EGD."

Whad he say? Whad he say?

This was jargon we call "hospitalese" which is the language medical professionals use because it's easier for us. We sometimes forget that non-medical folks don't understand it.

So, what did he really say?

An NG tube is a naso (nose) gastric (stomach) tube through the nose into the stomach to empty the stomach; it can be a life-saving device at times. You'll receive NPO which is English for the Latin "Nil per os" meaning nothing by mouth. We'll keep you on intravenous fluids into the vein to provide liquid until you can eat and drink again. The GI series (gastro-intestinal) is a group of X-rays of the stomach and intestines. An upper GI is a set of X-rays of the same organs, during which you drink radio opaque material. The BE is a barium enema in which the material is inserted in the rectum, providing X-rays of the lower intestine. The final possible test he is considering for you is the EGD which is an esophogastroduodenoscopy.

An esophogastroduodenoscopy (just to prove I can spell it again) consists of a tube from the mouth down the esophagus into the stomach (gastro), and duoden, the upper section of the small bowel, and enables the physician to look through the tube with a light, hence the word "oscopy." The physician can actually see into the stomach and the small intestine.

Isn't that a superb tongue twister—"esophogastroduodenoscopy"?

Perhaps another familiar example might be in order. Suppose the physician said "Your physical therapy treatments will be changed to bid from tid." He means changed to twice daily from three times daily. These are examples of how the jargon is frequently based on the original Latin. For example, *bid* is the shortened *bi diem* — *bi* is two in Latin and *diem* means day; hence, twice a day. Tid is derived from *tri diem* or three times a day.

The important thing is for you to ask for a translation if you don't understand what has been said. You will be more able to participate in making decisions about your care.

So, remember, whad he say?

Kay Erickson, RN, CCRN
Coupeville, Washington

BRING BACK THE DREAM LADY

Mrs. P was dying and she knew it. She took it all in stride, though. The nurses who cared for her found her quiet courage inspiring.

However, Mrs. P's pain kept her from sleeping. She had refused continuous drip morphine, so the nurses medicated her regularly, to prevent severe pain. They were successful for the most part, but her pain interrupted her sleep. She slept for two hours at the most. When I asked what she wanted most, she said, "Sleep. A little peaceful sleep."

I asked Mrs. P if she had ever tried hypnosis. She said no but that she would try anything.

When she said that she was as comfortable as possible in an armchair padded with pillows, we began. "Close your eyes, take a deep breath and hold it. Let it out and let your body relax. Feel yourself sinking down through the cushion of the chair. As you continue to breathe slowly and deeply, feel your muscles loosen and your body conform to the chair. Be aware of the seat of the chair supporting your weight and the back of the chair supporting your shoulders. Again, breathing slowly and deeply, allow yourself to become more and more relaxed.

"There are other sounds, but you hear my voice most distinctly. You will become more and more relaxed, more and more rested, more and more at peace. Time is slowing down and you begin to realize you have so-o much time. While you continue to breathe slowly and deeply, imagine yourself going to a peaceful place. You see how everything looks there. You may even hear sounds and notice smells. Realize how good it feels to be there. Stay there as long as you like. When you choose, come back and slowly open your eyes."

Quietly, I left the room. When she woke, she asked for the "dream lady." Mrs. P had slept for three hours and wanted another session.

Although there was nothing mysterious in what we did, she felt that there was something magical about her being able to sleep for so long. I found magic in easing her suffering and sharing her peace.

Kathleen Beyerman, RN, MSN, EdD
Cambridge, Massachusetts

(Reprinted with special permission from The American Journal of Nursing, September 1986 issue.)

LIFE IN HARRINGTON HALL

It was in about Martinmas time and the green leaves were a falling[1] when a group of girls, mainly from Minnesota, enrolled in the School of Nursing at the University of Minnesota — to take the five-year nurse training course. This was in 1940. Even then, the School of Nursing at Minnesota was highly respected.

Part of this group was destined to become a closely-knit clan of dear friends who, still today, 51 years later, meet to relive their earlier days.

For two years they studied on campus, living on or off campus, some commuting from home. Then came the assignment to training hospitals for the remaining three years. There were basically two choices — the University of Minnesota hospital or the Minneapolis General hospital, called "The General," perhaps affectionately. There was a definite preferential choice — they wanted University because Powell Hall, the nurses' residence, overlooked the Mississippi River, had a grand reception room and each girl had her own room. But they were assigned to General, being told they were assigned on an alphabetic basis. "It spelled the end of some friendships," recalled Virginia Purdy, "because the total involvement in work and study for the next three years somehow prevented us from seeing each other and now living so closely with others promoted the formation of new friendships, which consumed any free time we had."

Living quarters for nurses at The General were in an old building. The rooms were designed for one occupant but two were placed in each room because of space demands. They were quite spartan. A cot, a table, a chest of drawers and a window. Not much else. Joanne remembers that "soot came in through the opened window, making the room dirty. But this was still depression times so, for most of us, we were accustomed to doubling up, sharing small space at home, but, by comparison, with the lush U. of M. nursing quarters where we had expected to go, it was very disappointing." "Very drab and austere," says Helen Jurkovich. "We scavenged orange crates for bedside tables." There was one communal bathroom for each floor and one telephone. The phone was near the rumbling wire-cage old elevator and whoever was closest answered the ring. She would then bellow (do ladies "bellow"?) the name of the callee and everyone knew who was being called, occasionally for a date.

"The food was terrible," continues Helen. "Food was rationed and we had to turn in our ration books. I remember our first meal: mashed potatoes, cottage cheese, white bread, milk and cottage pudding. All white and tasteless, served family style and the bowl often nearly empty when it reached the last person. The doctors and interns had their own dining room and better food, so we circulated a petition in the dorm and sent a few students to the city council, since General was a city hospital then. Apparently they were met with compassion, for soon after a lovely new cafeteria was installed for all the staff and much better food was served. For this action we were called "the troublemakers."

"We developed a close camaradarie," Helen continued. "because we lived so closely, a situation that didn't seem to exist at other hospitals."

It wasn't a training popular with parents. One mother told her daughter that she definitely didn't want her to be a nurse — "working with all those people." It may not have been considered romantic but it certainly was exciting. "We had a wide array of clientele — very poor but also ordinary folks and even well-to-do on occasion. Firemen and police injured in line of duty were treated at General, plus all manner of accident victims, burns and explosions. All contagious diseases and all races. Being at General was far different from being at any other hospital, and therefore was more difficult. It was a rich and colorful experience and left me with more wisdom and compassion to all people."

Of course this was wartime. It was in 1942 when they went to The General. Pearl Harbor had occurred and men were in the service. The nurses eventually wore special uniforms and were called "cadet nurses," being members of the U.S. Cadet Nurse Corps. To entice more nurses into schools, the cadet nurse pay was increased to $20 a month, versus the intern pay of only $15 per month.

Since there was also such a need for nurses, in 1943 the hospital added four additional floors to the existing eight of the nurses' dorm. It was named Harrington Hall after The General's superintendent, Dr. Francis Harrington, probably a well-deserved recognition since Dr. Harrington was highly respected for greatly reducing deaths from tuberculosis in the city and "for giving the city one of the lowest infant and maternal death rates in the country."[2]

But life for the student nurses in General was a difficult assignment, consisting of huge workloads, long hours and continued classes through the University School of Nursing. Virginia remembers that "one of the first words that comes to mind regarding nurses' training was 'fatigue.' We were tired! For some students going to sleep at an early hour was impossible. They had a compelling need to stay up late to talk to others or to read to affirm that they were still human beings and not automatons. Losing sleep at night only meant more fatigue."

They were drilled to be neat, no nail polish, no perfume, no heavy makeup. White oxfords kept spotless and white cotton hose. Uniforms discreetly below the knees.

"We were on duty from 7 to 11 AM," says Joanne, "or 7 to 12 noon, allowing 30 minutes for lunch and then the streetcar ride to the campus for two or three hours of classes. We also had 'relief duty' instead of free evenings."

She continues: "And you didn't just leave if your work load were unfinished. You stayed to see that the evening 'cares' were done. We were also assigned to sharpening and cleaning IV equipment and needles, preparing everything for the autoclave in Sterile Supply. Remember, throw-away equipment is fairly new. We held rubber tubes together for nasal suction, sometimes using adhesive tape. The army and navy hospitals had priorities on rubber goods as well as access to the newly discovered miracle drugs. We had very little either sulfa or penicillin available for civilian use."

"We were no sooner assigned to The General and put to work than I had to be hospitalized as a patient," said Laura Donney. "I had some problems and couldn't even take part in my capping ceremony. I have always felt sorry about that."

"But," said someone, "you didn't miss much. All that happened was they gave each of us a square of cloth and told us how to fold it into our particular cap."

"Oh, yes, but how I loved my cap," said Evelyn Frey. "It was a symbol and I was proud of it. I think if I went back to work I'd like to wear it."

"Oh, no, they wouldn't let you," said someone else. "They don't do that today."

"But remember those strict rules — the hair couldn't touch the collar of the dress — and remember — did those starched uniforms really come to us like boards?" asked Virginia Purdy.

"Yes, they did," chorused all.

"How I remember our proby (probationary) years," said one of the group. Joanne remembered her first day: "I was working in a men's ward, going over charts at a desk, when another nurse told me to stand up quickly, because here came Doctor Jones and his entourage making rounds. We all knew he was a great stickler for details and arose for him. At that moment, I heard strange noises coming from a nearby patient's bed, which was surrounded by solid-sides to restrain him. My Lord, he was convulsing. "Grab the tongue blade," someone yelled. Afterwards, I knew there was a padded tongue depressor close to his bed but, remembering where they were stored, I ran to get one. I opened the door in a hurry—wrong door. I was in a closet. I went in, shut the door on myself and stayed there, hiding and shaking like a leaf, unable to come out."

"Be sure to write about Maxine," said Evelyn. "She was one of the original Northwest Airlines nurse-stewardesses when all the stewardesses had to be nurses." (For details of this interview, see "One of the First Nurse-Stewardesses" elsewhere in this book.)

But Harrington Hall doesn't exist anymore. The building had been used for years for other purposes, such as storage, and had to be destroyed to make way for progress.

In fact, while it was being demolished in 1989 Evelyn drove by the site and convinced a worker to save her some of the yellow exterior bricks as memorabilia of dear old Harrington Hall where she had become a nurse. Evelyn obtained them for the group, which kept them for doorstops and other uses. Joanne said those bricks "represent the heart and soul and blood and sweat of a great many young women who lived, worked, studied together. God bless them all, the patients, the students, the instructors, the grads on floor duty and the doctors and residents."

Helen summarizes: "We had remarkable experiences at General. We saw first hand patients injured from accidents, shootings, stabbings, explosions—and the violence of the weekends. General had its own ambulances and an intern always rode with the driver.

"The reasons we were so close—as a group—was all these rich experiences, dealing with all of mankind and often during great crises. We learned to respect all mankind, often society's outcasts were the most grateful for our caring. I felt profoundly changed to see the quality of care being provided these patients. The sickest patients got the most attention—and it's still that way at General's successor, Hennepin County Medical Center.

"Our experiences were more varied than at private hospitals. We cared for people with polio during the great epidemics, some patients being in iron lungs. Also with meningitis, diphtheria, tuberculosis, severe measles or chicken pox. We even had locked psychiatric wards and all manner of outpatient clinics.

"We were close because we lived together during those difficult war years. Boy friends were gone, news and letters were prized. We shared with each other our apprehensions about our experiences, our fears, joys, food from home, party clothes when someone's sweetheart came home on leave.

"It was a very unique and difficult experience, but profoundly changed my life. I became more tolerant, wiser, more sure of myself, and I think a better person."

Laura Donney, Rochester, MN
Evelyn Frey, Edina, MN
Helen Jurkovich, Minneapolis, MN
Joanne Murnane, Hastings, MN
Virginia Purdy, Minneapolis, MN

1. From "Barbara Allen" an old popular ballad, out of copyright protection.

2. (Minneapolis) Star-Tribune, February 2, 1990.

BETTY MADE IT TO THE SHOWER

When I was working in Seattle, I met Betty, a caring, dedicated nurse. She always went that extra mile to help the patient feel better. One day she got Mr. Hansen out of bed to use the toilet. He was a recovering alcoholic who hadn't been up is several days and was very weak. He had been on prolonged tube feeding which colored the characteristic ICU green. He also had a Foley catheter. As he slipped out of bed and was teetering on the brink of collapse, Betty noticed that his catheter was tugging on the bag still attached to the bed. She bent down with her head between the patient's legs to move the catheter bag. At that moment, poor Mr. Hansen tried so hard but couldn't hold it another second and he excreted on Betty's head. Betty yelled for help. We all came to her rescue with horror at the event that had just transpired. Mr. Hansen made it to the chair, Betty made it to the shower, and we made it to the lounge where we tried to control ourselves. The moral of the story — don't put your head in direct line with any patient's orifice.

Sherry J. Reynolds, RN, BS, CCRN
Cedar Hill, Texas

CAREFUL WITH THAT COLD STETHOSCOPE

In the spring semester of 1991 I accepted a position as clinical instructor at a nursing school. I was to monitor first semester, first year nursing students during their clinical rotation in the hospital and then have a two-hour post-conference the following day. We did this every week during the semester.

I had a quite varied but lively group, and we frequently had some interesting discussions. I thought that my eleven years of ICU nursing, coupled with lectures on different topics, would be adequate preparation for dealing with "green" nursing students and their many questions, until I met George.

George was very excited about becoming a nurse, and his enthusiasm was infectious. He was always interested in new procedures and enjoyed discussing what he had learned the previous week, when we had our post-conference.

One day in post-conference I was teaching the students how to listen to heart and lung sounds. George began to relate his latest learning experience on the subject, but he chose to listen to areas of the body which nurses don't auscultate.

He said, "You know, the best way to learn things is by doing them. I came home the other day after school and I still had my stethoscope around my neck. Well, my roommate was home . . ."

"Yes?"

". . . and he was lying on the bed . . ."

"Yes?"

". . . and he didn't have any clothes on."

"Uh, huh." At this point I was beginning to wonder where this story was headed.

"Well, I just decided to practice listening to his lungs and, well,

I listened to . . . uh . . . well, have you ever listened to any-one's . . . uh . . . testicles?"

All of my students erupted in laughter and I started to give my-self a mental pep talk about my ability to control the class and get the conversation on a higher plane. So I very calmly said, "No, George, I can't say that I have."

"Well, it sounded like little bowel sounds."

My students were still giggling and I was still silently coaching myself on what I could say to get the conversation back on track. At that point I thought of my experiences listening to my asthmatic son's lungs and related that sometimes I could hear referred bowel sounds in the chest area. Unfortunately, it didn't stop the direction of the discussion, which was headed for the gutter.

Again, George had comments to make.

"Oh, but that's not all. Next I put my stethoscope on his penis and you know what it sounded like? Like a heart beat."

Now, all of my students except one began to howl with laughter. Mae, my studious Oriental student, always known for her power of concentration and inquiring mind, then asked with all seriousness, "Is that because of all of the extra blood flow?"

Needless to say, at that point, even I was laughing. The students were roaring and I have no memory of what happened the rest of the class.

I told my friends at work about my experiences with the students. We all had a good laugh and decided that we should add a new sec-tion to our assessment flow sheet. We are going to call it "Scrotum Sounds."

Susan Neibel, RN, BSN, CCRN
Dallas, Texas

THE GROUND FLOOR'S CONNECTED
TO THE FIRST FLOOR

I work in the ICU of a large hospital which is connected to a medical school at the ground level. One day I was taking care of a patient in the unit who was ordred to have a special blood flow study of her brain. Usually, these studies could be done at the hospital but, for some reason, it was determined that she needed the expertise of the staff at the medical school.

I gathered all of the equipment needed for the transport, including her IVs, IV pumps and poles, the emergency drug box, the transportable monitor, her chart, and the oxygen tank connected to her nasal cannula. I carefully placed all of these items in the bed with my very large patient.

The hospital transport was experienced in taking patients to and from the two buildings and, even though neither she nor I was familiar with where the brain blood flow study lab was located, we naively felt that we could get there easily with the help of the lab director. He had called to tell us his beeper number so when we were ready to leave he would be available to meet us on the ground floor.

Unfortunately, he didn't tell us which ground floor.

The ground floors of each building are not on the same level because the basement of the hospital is connected to the ground floor of the school, while the ground floor of the hospital is connected to the first floor of the medical school. Thus one does not just walk from ground floor to ground floor when changing buildings.

We left the ground floor of the hospital to the point where it ended and the medical school began. The director of the lab wasn't there because he was on the ground floor of the med school. However, the transporter felt she could get us to our goal, having been there once before. I reluctantly agreed and we continued our journey.

We wandered until we came to a set of elevators. We had been told that the brain blood flow lab was on the sixth floor, but we had not been told that only one of the many medical school elevators could accommodate a patient bed.

We had already tried two different sets of elevators when we came upon another, which appeared larger. I put the side rails down on the bed to get it into the elevator and squeezed in myself. The bed still had about six inches sticking out in the hallway so we decided to try elsewhere. I was already beginning to sweat from all of the hassle and exertion, when one of the wheels of the bed fell in the crack between the elevator and the floor. The bed began to tip over onto me and the patient started to fall out. I was doing my best to keep her in the bed and to prevent myself from being flattened like a pancake.

Then the normal saline hooked to her nasal cannula spilled over into the cannula tubing and up into her nose. She began to fling her arms wildly because she was already confused and didn't know why she had a sudden case of extreme post-nasal drip.

At this point I could contain myself no longer and began to verbally plot the death of the resident who had ordered this %&$#& test.

The transporter began to yell for help and three large men with weightlifter muscles appeared from nowhere. They physically lifted the bed out of the crack and pointed us to yet another elevator.

We proceeded up to the sixth floor, stupidly thinking that we had reached our destination, only to find ourselves in the OB-GYN section of the med school. Everyone looked at us as if we had lost our minds, which we were definitely in danger of doing at that point. Finally, at the brink of frustration and physical exhaustion, I remembered that I had the lab director's beeper number. I called my charge nurse who got in touch with him. He eventually found us and took us to his lab.

The test and travel time getting to and from the lab should have taken only one and a half hours. It took us three and one half that day. We wandered like Moses looking for the Promised Land for over 40 minutes. A friend who heard my story had to tell me why Moses and the Israelites had wandered for forty years before reaching their destination. It was because even back then, men still never asked for directions. And until that day, I didn't think I had that characteristic in common with them.

Susan Neibel, RN, BSN, CCRN
Dallas, Texas

A BABY'S CRY

It was late Friday night and I was working the 11 PM to 7:30 AM shift on the labor and delivery unit. I had been doing this nursing specialty for over 15 years and still enjoyed each new life that I helped bring into the world. My particular patient's name was Sarah. Sarah and I knew each other because I had helped deliver her first child, a girl, 2 years ago. There is something special about the relationship a woman in labor has with her nurse.

The time was 12:28 AM Saturday and Sarah was having difficulty in the progression of her labor. The doctor, a general practitioner, had ordered an abdominal x-ray for the presenting part of the fetus. Sarah and I prepared to go downstairs to the main floor to the x-ray department. We were on the 5th floor of the hospital. I talked to her mother and told her what we were going to do and invited her to go with us. Sarah's husband was not with her through this labor and delivery. I really don't know why, it was just one of those times when there was no man with the woman. Sarah's mother said she was tired and would wait in the lounge and rest till we got back.

I covered Sarah with a thermal blanket and pushed her through the doors to the elevator and pushed the button to the main floor. She and I had a nice talk during our ride on the elevator. I tried to explain what was going on with the labor and why the doctor wanted this x-ray. I pushed her off the elevator and down the corridor to the radiology department where the technician was waiting. I helped Sarah move from the labor cart onto the x-ray table. I was getting her as comfortable as possible when the bag of waters ruptured and out of her vagina flew the umbilical cord. I stood there in what I know as shock and panic on my face. The cord was long. It was past her knees and she was a tall woman, about 5 ft. 10 in.

The x-ray technician looked at me with fright and I started to throw orders at him. I put on a sterile rubber glove and told Sarah what had happened and that I was going to hold her baby's head up out of the way. I inserted my whole hand and Sarah cried—no screamed—in pain. I tried to console her and still keep my wits about me. I told the technician to call the labor and delivery department and tell them that I had a prolapsed cord and to get help. The technician left us to make the phone call. Sarah and I got ourselves under control and I laid the cord on my arm so that I could see the pulsation in the cord. I could feel the cord laying between my fingers and coming down the palm of my hand. This baby was alive and I was going to see to it that it stayed that way. I had lost a baby about a month before from a very short prolapsed cord.

The x-ray technician came back into the room and told me he had made the call and they were calling a surgeon. We were to go to surgery. I told the technician to cover us up as best he could with thermal blanket and help us to surgery which was just around the corner from radiology. The cord was still pulsating. I could feel it and see it.

I really think that was the longest walk I had ever taken. I continued to reassure Sarah that everything was under control and the baby was okay. I prayed to God that He help me through this one. God and I do a lot together in my nursing. I know that He is the one who helped me keep it together in trying times such as this one. We went through the door of the surgical suite and the operating crew came to life. I looked at the clock and it was 12:50 AM. My hand and arm were starting to hurt from holding the baby up out of the pelvis. Her contractions were getting stronger and closer together. She began to cry and so did I.

By this time, my hand and arm were really hurting. My head was under the covers and the tears came to my eyes from the pain I was feeling and also I think from the fear I was feeling inside. Again, I tried to reassure Sarah that the baby was okay and that I was doing okay too. I told her that my hand was hurting but not to worry because I was going to save this baby's life with her help. I know that she was hurting more than any of us with the strength of her contractions which were now every 2-3 minutes and very strong. I was trying to encourage her not to do any pushing, although I know the urge must have been great with my entire hand in her vagina and on her baby's head.

I looked at the clock and it was 1:20 AM when the doctor finally walked in. I thought he would never get there. He said "What you got, Anna?" I told him with tears running down my cheeks that I had a live baby with a pulsating umbilical cord laying on my arm. He replied, "Are you sure that baby's alive?" I said, "YES, now get in there and help me!" He mumbled something about "If I had been told it was a live baby I would have hurried." He started to scrub and then said "the hell with it" and gowned and gloved. He told me that when he said to take my hand out to do just that. I said okay but told him that I had no feeling in my hand and my arm hurt really bad.

The anesthetist gave Sarah a general anesthetic and she fell asleep. After draping, an incision was made. Again the doctor asked me how the baby was doing and I looked at the cord and said okay. He made an incision into the uterus and put his finger in. He felt my fingers and told me to remove my hand. I tried. I couldn't. I screamed at him "I can't." He began to cut the uterus with a scalpel and asked me if he had cut my fingers. I told him I didn't know because my entire hand and arm were paralyzed by now. He reached into the womb and pulled out a crying 10 pound 14 ounce healthy baby boy. I just sobbed. I was so relieved to hear that cry. Some of the OR staff helped remove my hand and the doctor pushed on it from his side. When I took off the sterile glove I noticed that my finger tips had been cut. I only had two finger tips that were cut but not bad, no stitches were required.

When he was in the nursery and I knew that he was going to be all right I went into the nurses lounge in labor and delivery and sat down and held my swollen hand and arm. My head nurse came over and put some ice on my hand. She sat down beside me and told me that I had done a nice job and got up and left. I sat there for a while going over the events of the night and said a little prayer to thank God for being there for me once again. I knew that down deep I had kept it together in one of the most stressful situations of my career.

Today, I look back on that delivery and thank God that He and I saved a life of what may be the president of this grand country. By the way I did receive a commendation for saving a life. To me the cry I heard was enough.

Anna Hines, RN, BSHA
Altoona, IA

INDEX

NURSE

NURSE